What Reviewers Say About
# *Look Like A Winner After 50*

"[Peddicord's] book offers mature women much more than advice about cosmetics, hairstyles and wardrobe. It suggests that feeling beautiful fosters a positive attitude and a better self-concept, important to women at any age."
*– The Denver Post Active Times magazine*
Denver, CO

"For women who've forgotten the basics, *Look Like A Winner* offers a refresher course...a jumpstart in updating their style....For every woman who's reached 50 and beyond, here's a reminder that birthdays don't count but she still does."
*– Rocky Mountain News*
Denver, CO

"*Look Like A Winner After 50* is fun to read because the reader can apply every bit of it to herself."
*– The Tribune*
Oklahoma City, OK

"Everything in this book seems to work hand in hand to make you look as good as you feel and feel as good as you look."
*– The Spring Lake News*
Spring Lake, NC

"Wonderful book...well put together. We are pleased to have a copy in our library."
*– HOPEline Director, My Image After Cancer*
Alexandria, VA

"Women over 50...will like Peddicord's common sense and affirming approach. She reminds women that age is no barrier to looking and feeling dynamic and alive, and that they are their best fashion advisors."
*– The Dialog*
Wilmington, DE

*Look Like A Winner After 50* received a Silver Award, Media/Books category, in the 1996 National Mature Media Awards Program. This program, presented by the Mature Market Resource Center in Illinois, recognizes the nation's finest advertising, marketing and educational materials designed and produced for older adults.

More than 1,000 entries were judged by a distinguished panel of mature market experts from across the United States for overall excellence of design, content, creativity and relevance to the senior market. This third edition has been enhanced to be an even more helpful and enjoyable reading experience.

"Today's 50+ woman is not waiting for life to roll by, she is grabbing and squeezing it for all it's worth. My publications explain the practical and proven solutions to looking her best for the roles she plays no matter what age or size she is."

*– Jo Peddicord*
author, nationally syndicated
columnist and speaker.

# LOOK LIKE A WINNER
# AFTER 50
## WITH CARE, COLOR & STYLE

by
Jo Peddicord

GOLDEN ASPEN PUBLISHING

Published by:
Golden Aspen Publishing
Post Office Box 370333
Denver, CO 80237-0333, U.S.A.
Fax (303) 694-0737, E-mail GAPub@aol.com

**Publisher's Cataloging in Publication**
*(Prepared by Quality Books Inc.)*
Peddicord, Jo.
   Look like a winner after 50 : with care, color and style / by Jo Peddicord; Jim Ayers, editor; Paul Koroshetz and Bobbi Shupe, illustrations. — 3rd ed.
   p. cm.
   Includes biographical references and index.
   ISBN 0-9654434-0-X
   1. Beauty, Personal.  2. Cosmetics.  3. Color in clothing.
4. Middle aged women—Health and hygiene.
I. Title.
RA778.P316 1997        646.7'042
                                  96-79098
                                  QB196-40199
3rd edition, completely revised
10  9  8  7  6  5  4  3  2  1

# My Sincere Thanks To

Production:
**Harald Prommel**, National Writers Press, Denver, CO

Illustrations:
**Paul Koroshetz** and **Bobbi Shupe**

Editing:
**Jim Ayers**, Criscadian Editorial Services, Denver, CO

Photography including cover:
**Michael Edwards**, Maxwell Studios Inc., Denver, CO

**Betty Reed**, Denver, CO, interviewed in Chapter 5, *Erasing the Wrinkles,* her photo is on page 175.

**Dr. Richard G. Asarch, Dr. Darryl Burns, Dr. Donald L. Finks, Dr. Robert Hoehn, Lois Tschetter Hjelmstad, Dr. George M. Lacy, Dr. Douglas A. McKinnon, Dr. Barbara Reed, Madelyn Stengel, Treva Stutzman,** all in Denver, CO and **Dr. Linda Fang,** Lafayette, CA for their generosity in helping me get the facts.

To the kind and courageous women I interviewed for Chapter 10, *Restoring a Positive Image After Mastectomy and Ileostomy,* for wanting to help with sage advice.

Jo Peddicord

# Dedication

This book is dedicated to women who have spent most of their lives nurturing others in homes, schools, colleges, universities, shops, stores, offices, industries, professions, institutions, and organizations of every kind in every country and who now recognize the need to nurture themselves.

# Contents

# Introduction

Looking like a winner after midlife can happen only when we let go of old concepts, embrace new ones, and refuse to be intimidated by the years. It can happen only when we let positive, promising and recreative concepts replace the outdated attitudes that say beauty is only for younger women. The women in my "Magic of Makeup" classes have learned that a winning look is a matter not of youth but of desire, caring and the intelligent use of color and style.

Jean arrived late to one of these classes and hurried as fast as her cane and body allowed to the last chair. "I need all the help I can get," she panted. Her husband waited in the doorway, saw her settled, then left. Jean looked around at everyone and breathlessly apologized for being late. "I really do need some help," she repeated, squeezing out a self-conscious smile. There was a ripple of sympathetic chuckling and the women nodded in agreement. They needed it, too.

Jean had a life-threatening disease that caused a prednisone hump on her back and a fleshy dewlap under her throat. She missed her graceful ballerina figure of many years ago, but still had a dramatic and impressive face, framed by white curly hair peppered with black. Her large, dark eyes flashed intelligently as she concentrated on every word. We talked about the why's and how's of applying makeup – the "trade" secrets that camouflage wrinkles and bring out ageless beauty. At the end of the class Jean asked for a personal consultation.

1

In her home I showed her how to maintain a healthy complexion and how to apply makeup artfully. Her husband, who had suggested the class, watched the transformation. Afterward, he exclaimed, "You look fantastic! Let's go out and celebrate!" The same week she went to a bridge party where for the first time in years, she was complimented on how good she looked. She not only looked lovely, she felt lovelier.

We consciously or unconsciously associate beauty with youth, but true beauty is ageless. Once we accept that, it is natural and appropriate to look as good as we want to.

Many women never think of themselves as attractive. They have been put down so subtly and convincingly that they unconsciously accept themselves as unattractive instead of challenging a derogatory remark or considering it mistaken. Too often we accept critical opinions without questioning them.

Critics ask, "Why all this fuss about beauty or glamour?" Granted, appearance should never be more important than what we say or do, but this is a visual society. Beauty is important. It is pleasant, soothing to the senses and inspires joy. That is why we enjoy gardens, hike in the mountains, walk in the park, listen to concerts, browse through art museums, hang pictures in our homes.

Plastic surgeon Dr. Maxwell Maltz wrote in his book, *Psycho-Cybernetics*, that self-esteem is as necessary to the spirit as food is to the body. Consequently, beauty, glamour, style – whatever you want to call it – is essential in our maturing years. When a woman creates her best appearance, she helps herself to overcome some of the loneliness and rejection she may feel.

Most societies see the age-etched face on men as masculine, even macho. On women, it is old. This is beginning to change. Care and makeup take years off the face and replace "aged" with "ageless," elevating how we feel about ourselves.

One over-50 woman told me she didn't need makeup because she wasn't dating anymore. This harkens back to teenage years when a date was THE most important event. Glamour is much more than a means to attract romance. It is a practical, personal necessity that enhances what nature gave us and shows respect for the person we are. When you can look in the mirror and think, "Not bad! I look good, even if I do say so," you will walk taller with a happier step. *That is the point.* Image reinforcement gives us a better self-concept and an edge in career pursuits, personal relationships – in all activities.

A nurse in a large metropolitan hospital told me her patients react to the way she looks. When she had a caring appearance *with* makeup, they were cooperative and cheerful. When she looked ordinary, they complained and were cantankerous. A similar message came from a school teacher. When she wore color on her face, she had fewer disciplinary problems. Right or wrong, the patients and students sensed that the nurse and teacher cared more about them when their appearance was better than "ordinary."

EVERYONE enjoys seeing a lovely woman. One Sunday morning my seventy-plus mother was leaving her home as a young man walked by. He glanced at her and suddenly stopped to say, "My, you look lovely!" Mother was astounded. No one had told her she looked "lovely" since my father died many years before. This compliment from a stranger brightened her whole day. Until then, she had been too focused on wrinkles and plumpness to recognize her ageless beauty.

In her book, *Always Beautiful,* Kaylan Pickford said that advertising conditions us to believe there is only one age that women are beautiful, our "golden age" begins in the teens and ends in the 30s. The truth is age is not a qualifying or determining factor of beauty. Just as an artist uses color to embellish a plain canvas, so we can create a colorful, appealing image.

The 1990 census shows that women over 45 constitute more than one-third of the female population of the United States. The industry has noticed. Publications on fashion and style are offering more information for our age group, much more than a decade ago. They are beginning to feature more mature women in their catalogues and brochures. Look at any audience during a fashion show and you will see that it is primarily women over 45. It is no wonder that the applause is hearty when they see one of their peers modeling clothing that is appropriate for them.

Although nearly all women over 40 wear eye glasses of some kind, how many times have you seen women past midlife in advertisements for glasses? Even periodicals geared to the fifty-plus market seldom have fifty-plus women in their optical ads. Fortunately, advertisers are improving their focus and beginning to recognize where the majority of their market is and what our needs are.

If the media has been slow to change, it may only be mirroring our acceptance of mediocrity. Many women are reticent about a spiffy appearance, one that says "fun." Has the absence of advertisements with beautiful mature women brainwashed us into thinking we are too old for beauty? It has taken us a long time to develop a special inner beauty. It's now time to encourage that beauty on the outside as well. Using only 15 percent of the information in this book will help you select suitable makeup, fashions and hair styles that do just that. This attractive new look will boost your morale and bring about a more positive outlook. The positive feeling is crucial and powerful. Sometimes we have to struggle to hold on to it, but once we discover that it flows from common sense, we will never surrender to negativity.

In *The Allure Book*[1], Julie Davis writes, "Thinking positively is step one. Projecting this positive energy through body language is step two. This means acting confident even if you don't yet feel it: head held high, shoulders straight, eyes interested. If you don't believe in the power of having an aura of confidence, take a walk along any busy avenue. Look at the faces of the people around you. Those who are smiling and projecting positive feelings are attractive. Those who have unpleasant expressions and downcast postures make you look the other way."

If you were content in the negative nest of "I can't" or "I'm not," you wouldn't be reading this book. Chances are you have been nurturing people most of your life. There is nothing wrong with that, but now expand your caring. It is time to nurture you.

> Thinking positive and maintaining
> an upbeat appearance
> brightens your life and is encouraging to
> family, friends and associates.

# 1

# The Magic of Color

"Color enriches the world and
our perception of it; a colorless
world is almost unimaginable."
— *Color* by Marshall Edition Ltd.[1]

At the beginning of a makeup class, two women complained about the rude treatment they had received in a restaurant:

"Why, I was treated as a non-person!"

"Yes, that happened to me, too," the other one chimed in.

"How did you look that day?" I asked.

"Oh, just about the way I do now, I guess."

"Did you smile when you were talking to the waiter?"

"Well, I don't know. Probably not. I haven't been feeling very well lately. What difference does that make?"

"All the difference in the world. When you look your best and smile, people treat you better."

What people see tells them about the person you are, and color plays a quiet but dynamic role in forming that impression. Another influence, our smile, colors the personality just as effectively as rainbow hues on face and figure color the body. The combination of an attractive, colorful appearance and a smile says, "I care – I care about you, and I care about me."

Color is to us what sunshine is to a day. Color makes us look younger or older, rested or tired, thinner or heavier, lovely or dowdy. It magnifies inner beauty.

Throughout history outstanding women have ingeniously combined stunning colors with fashion and cosmetics. Their motivations were both personal and societal. Over 20 centuries have passed, but Cleopatra's high style and makeup – the dramatically defined eyes – left an indelible impression that still lives on.

Elizabeth I, who ruled England from age 25 to her death at 69, was always seen in elegant coiffures, makeup, jewels, and vibrant colors in gem-studded gowns. Her unrivaled image and personality contributed to her undisputed superiority in the 1500s. The royal court and admiring crowds were enthralled with her majesty and poise. A biographer relates that even when she was dying, she was dressed royally *with* makeup. She knew the importance of image. Today's modern women are equally aware of the impact of image and are doing the same with a more simplified style.

## *The Psychology of Color*

In *The Art of Color,* Johannes Itten wrote, "Colors are forces, radiant energies that affect us positively or negatively, whether we are aware of it or not."[2]

These color forces vibrate warmth, energy, tranquility, and their opposites, which, in turn, affect health, comfort, happiness and safety.[3] Because yellow is the most luminous color in the spectrum, has the highest visibility, and is conspicuous under all lighting conditions, it is used in over 20 traffic signs. The capacity of color to influence human behavior has been proven by extensive research. From industrial, government, and armed services facilities to hospitals, schools and businesses – people react to the cheery or drab color combinations in their environment.

"We do know that people feel happier when surrounded by certain colors," *The Standard Textbook for Professional Esthetiticians** states. "Some color experts say that the colors we use in our homes are definite indications of personality traits. For example, people who surround themselves with cool colors, such as green and blue, may be expressing their desire for peace and tranquility. People who use an abundance of bright colors, such as red, orange, and yellow, are usually people who love gaiety and are outgoing....We may not realize to what extent we are affected by color, but when you awaken on a dull, gloomy morning, you probably will reach for something bright and cheerful to wear."[3]

When you have aches and pains, that's the time to wear bright, lively color, because the body responds to colors that suggest vitality. The psychological healing power of color is a major consideration in the interior decoration of hospitals and care facilities. Color-healing, an ancient science, is described in Faber Birren's book, *Color Psychology and Color Therapy*. Because Birren has extensively researched and written about color science, large and small corporations and governmental facilities worldwide have requested his advice on color environments that make for better safety and productivity.[4]

Some people feel a definite discomfort with certain colors. They can even have color allergies. During the brief color analysis for each woman in makeup classes, the color that gets the most negative response is orange. One woman physically withdrew from it and wanted no part of it. Only a small percentage liked or looked good in orange. No such reaction occurred with red, misty green and peach that everyone liked.

Colors inspire emotional responses. Certain ones "feel" comfortable, others don't. Trust your intuition. Wear only the colors that kindle confidence and brighten your countenance. When you wear colors that attract compliments, you can't help feeling happier.

---

* Reprinted by permission of Milady Publishing Company from the publication, *Standard Textbook for Professional Estheticians,* by Joel Gerson.

Be adventurous and try different colors. It's exciting to find a new shade that is positively smashing. Perhaps you never thought of wearing it. Perhaps you wore it 30 years ago and now have the ridiculous idea that you are too old for it. If it beautifies, wear it.

## *The Color Personality*

Each of us has a distinctive color personality. It is composed of all the shades in the rainbow, but in a one-of-a-kind combination. Examine the colors in your skin, hair and eyes. These, plus their relating and complementary colors, comprise your color personality and are your best choices for anything you wear or put in your environment.

The skin of all ethnics contains the three primary colors – yellow, red and blue. Everyone's skin has yellow plus melanin, the darkening agent. The red and blue blood supply bring in the other two primary colors. These physiological elements combine and create a predominance of either a blue/pink or a yellow coloring in the pigmentation. This combination is called the undertones Skin that has a preponderance of blue/pink is said to have a cool undertone. Skin that has a preponderance of yellow has a warm undertone. This pertains to the many complexions of the human race. Here is a sampling of cool and warm undertones as they relate to race:

| Race | Cool Undertones | Warm Undertones |
|---|---|---|
| White | blue-pink | peach, coral |
| Black | charcoal, ashen gray | golden |
| Hispanic, Oriental, and Asian | olive | golden |

The colors that look best on you consist of either warm or cool components. Whatever makeup you use, whatever clothes you wear, will either compliment or conflict with your unique combination of undertones.

Using the seasonal concept, here are examples of warm and cool colors that will give you a fairly good idea of what colors and temperature attracts your interest:

Warm, Vibrant (Spring): orange-red, bright yellow, kelly green, royal blue

Warm, Earthy (Fall): rust, bittersweet red, moss green, purple

Cool, Pastel (Summer): watermellon, very pale yellow, misty green, lavender, powder blue

Cool, Vivid (Winter): blue-red, a deep yellow, navy blue, forest green

## Color Analysis Get Help or Do Your Own

You are probably thinking, "Fine, but how do I know what colors are warm or cool, and which ones look good on me?" If your skin tends to burn when exposed to the sun, your skin tones are apt to be cool. But, if you tan easily, they are warm.

A color analysis by a qualified professional is worth the time and money, especially if color has always been a problem. They may be listed in the yellow pages of your phone book under "Color Consultants." In some women the physiological difference between the warm and cool undertones is borderline. She may have a combination of both tones that causes color confusion. A qualified and experienced analyst eliminates this.

Besides being fun and educational, a color sitting opens the mind to a broad range of enticing, new shades. The client is given fans, booklets or folders suitable for the individual, containing anywhere from 20 to 200 shades. Not all shades will be good for you. They are guidelines and excellent time savers when you are shopping for clothes, makeup, household decorations and furnishings anything pertaining to color.

A good analyst guarantees satisfaction and will give referrals. If you have had an analysis and don't feel right about the recommended colors, the analyst should offer another session to resolve the question, refund the cost or refer you to another analyst.

You can do your own color analysis. Here are some choices:

- With the help of a consultant or salesperson, apply two shades of foundation or base, one with a blue base (cool), such as rose or natural beige, and one with a yellow base (warm), such as golden beige. Apply where you have no makeup or the inside of your wrist. The shade that blends naturally with your skin is the right one. If you have difficulty deciding under store lights, compare the shades in daylight.

- Spend half an hour in a fabric shop during their slow time. Find the table with solid red colors. Pick one that is blue-red (cool) and one that is orange-red (warm). If you cannot make this distinction, ask a sales person. Which one, the blue-red or orange-red casts a pleasing reflection on your face? The right color gives the face clarity, the wrong one makes the face look drawn and older, sometimes even haggard. Observe the different shades of black – the flat or dull black (cool) versus the richer (warm) black; stark white (cool) versus creamy (warm) white. Then, use this comparison with other fabric colors. What is your reaction to each shade? Do you like it? Ask for swatches of the fabrics that you think look exceptionally good on you.

- Some women have successfully made a color decision by draping the fabrics on the lower half of their arms and noticing the reaction of the color against their skin.

- Your intuitive preference is a strong indicator. Examine the clothing in your closet. If you see lots of pastels or deep, jewel tones, you have a preference for cool shades. If there are bright, vibrant or earthy colors, you favor the warm ones. Your most flattering shades are either in the warm dominant or cool dominant family of colors.

The blues, purples, blacks and whites that are in the warm family are made with more yellow in the manufacturing process. The same colors in the cool family have more blue or pink in the mix. Train your eye to see the difference. Neutral colors have a balance of both the yellow and blue/pink bases. This is a simplistic explanation of a very complicated and technical process.

When it comes to jewelry, gold is considered warm and silver, cool. Usually, women with warm undertones wear gold and those with cool undertones wear silver. Some women have no preference and wear both. When it looks good against the skin, it works.

## *Color and Makeup*

The magical colors of makeup transform an ordinary, plain-looking face into one that is vital, youthful and attractive. The idea behind the *Pygmalion* and *My Fair Lady* stories, that a nondescript woman can be changed into a beautiful one, is not fiction. It has enduring significance. The mature woman can look five to 10 years younger with the intelligent use of color, particularly on the face. The cells in the skin that produce pigmentation decrease as we age; the skin gets paler. That's why makeup is more important after 50 and why we wear more, not less.

No matter how well makeup is applied, if the colors are wrong for the tones in the skin, the result is unbecoming. We analyze each woman's color personality before individual application in my makeup classes. Using both warm and cool shades in two or three color groups, such as the reds, purples, and greens, we hold them under the chin of each person to see how they react with the complexion. Someone will say, "That color turns her face grey." When we try the opposite temperature, they will remark, "Yes, that lightens up her face and she looks much better."

Comparing yellow-based and blue-based colors with the complexion is decisive. Colors appropriate for a person's skin tones minimize the lines and wrinkles and clarify the complexion. Wrong colors accentuate shadows or blotches and make the skin look pale, sallow or dull.

If your undertones are cool, you want lip and blush shades related to the orchids, roses, mauves, or blue-reds. If they are warm, look at the corals, apricots, bronzes, or orange-reds. Some cosmetic manufacturers make selection easier by coding their products as "warm" or "cool."

Linda attended one of my classes. She had a flawless, alabaster complexion with Grecian contours. The beauty potential was so apparent that women couldn't help asking her why she didn't wear makeup. She responded, "I don't know how, and I'm afraid of looking unnatural."

With my help, she started with foundation and applied soft colorings feature-by-feature, each step unveiling her loveliness. When she finished, she was amazed at the beautiful woman who smiled back in the mirror. She never thought of herself that way, and the transformation was almost more than she could believe.

## Color and Clothing

Color is as important as style. It may be an unconscious decision, but most of us won't wear even a stunning designer fashion if it's the wrong color. It just hangs in the closet and we wonder why we ever bought it. When shopping, you can save time and money by looking first for color, then style. Once your eye is trained to recognize your best colors, you quickly know the clothing colors that will work and those that won't.

The colors worn around the throat and shoulders reflect up to the face. They should be flattering light or bright shades.

Dark colors, such as navy and black, worn around the face bring out facial shadows, wrinkles and lines. One way to soften this effect is to tuck a chiffon or silk scarf with white-infused pastels into the V-neck or jewel neckline of jackets, sweaters or dresses.

Using monochromatic colors (shades in the same family), such as a pale pink blouse with dark pink slacks or a pearl grey sweater with a dark grey skirt, is figure-friendly and pleasing to the eye. Bold, bright colors look best with neutrals, for example, a fuschia, red or cobalt blue sweater over white wool slacks. Common neutrals are white, gray, beige, brown, navy and black.

Brilliant colors belong in your wardrobe when they fit your personality and comfort zone. An Italian-born grandmother said she was so happy to live in the United States. In Italy she would be expected to wear the dark blues and blacks that are traditionally proper for women past forty. Here, she can wear the brighter shades that make her feel alive.

## Total Color Harmony

Total color harmony in all facets of appearance results in classic style. Everything works together. This means that all the colors we wear in clothes, accessories, and makeup are blue/pink-based (cool) or yellow-based (warm). They don't fight or conflict with each other. To see this principle in action, browse through fashion magazines and analyze the color plates.

## Red Is Special

Red is dynamic, the queen of all colors. This primary color demands attention and deserves special mention. For the woman over 50, its high-energy hue is more effective in soft, matte fabrics, such as wool gabardine and jersey, rather than in shiny ones. If you want to soften its exciting impact, combine it with white, for example, a red blazer over a white knit sweater or a red shirt with a beige skirt.

Red comes in many shades. To get all of the advantages of this striking color be sure the color of your makeup and jewelry, and maybe shoes, do not fight with your red dress or suit. At a Sunday afternoon tea that I attended, a woman wore an attractive Chinese red suit. It was orange-red, but her lip color was a bluish magenta that "pinched" her mouth, blanched out her face, and clashed with her suit. A matching orange-red lip color would have softened facial lines and harmonized with the suit. Because red is eye-catching, take care that your cheek and lip colors perfectly match and cooperate with the red in your clothing. The same goes for earrings. Or, match them to the gold or silver of the buttons.

## The Focal Point of Appearance

The face is the focal point of our image. Makeup colorings are no longer superficial. They are essential to the ageless concept. If the makeup beautifies, the hair color flatters, and you put on a smile, you could wear a burlap bag (the right color, of course!) and attract the admiring eye of a passerby!

# 2

# The Basics

"I'm tired of all this nonsense about
beauty being only skin-deep.
That's deep enough. What do you
want—an adorable pancreas?"
— Jean Kerr, 1960[1]

"What is the first thing you notice about a person?" I asked
one of my makeup classes. One woman surprised us by saying
she noticed a person's tummy first. She appraised women starting at the midsection! The most popular response is: The face –
it triggers that important first impression while peripheral
vision takes in the rest. Facial attractiveness starts with a cared-
for complexion.

The lifestyle of many women adversely affect their skin –
from health abusers, such as the sun, poor eating habits,
alcohol, and cigarettes, to stress, work environment, travel, and
pollution. These and other factors make skin problems
common. So, it is imperative to nourish and care for the skin
regularly. Cosmetic companies are continuing to develop excellent skin care products that meet the needs of every woman.

Slow the aging process of the skin by observing the
following:

- Use sunscreen when you sunbathe. Keep the face and
  throat shaded. Excessive sun exposure causes brown spots,
  weakens the elastic fibers, and damages the underlying
  collagen. It can also penetrate the thin layer around the
  eyes, causing pigment changes and dark under-eye circles.

- To prevent facial tension lines, fit into your schedule stress-relieving outlets – walking, sports, exercise, etc., or aromatherapy. Aromatherapy is the use of essential oils from plants for therapeutic purposes. Example: the scent of lavender oil calms.

- Avoid the skin-aging habits of frowning, squinting, scowling, and excessive smoking or alcohol. The last two dehydrate and deplete nutrients from the body. Nicotine constricts blood vessels, diminishing the flow of blood to the skin. Inhaling eventually causes deep lines around the lips.

- Use an effective cleansing routine that includes masking/ exfoliating and moisturizing. It helps to reduce the visibility of lines.

- Get as much sleep as you require, usually six to eight hours. Lack of it shows up on the face.

## Good Ingestion

Healthier skin is one advantage of good eating and drinking patterns. The skin is nourished by nutrients in the bloodstream. A well-balanced diet is insurance for healthy skin. Cut down or eliminate sugar and salt. Eat plenty of fresh fruits and vegetables, nuts, seeds, some fats, and drink as much water as you can. Water detoxifies the system by flushing out impurities. *Don't wait until you are thirsty* or, you may be on your way to dehydration (lack of moisture in the system). Warning signs are fatigue, loss of appetite, heat intolerance, impatience, and dizziness. If water is boring, add pineapple bits, a lemon wedge, an orange slice, a sliver of kiwi or a splash of cranberry juice for a tart twist.

Dehydration is a primary cause of dry, lined skin. Oranges are excellent for skin because they are 80% water and contain vitamin C that is essential to collagen production. Collagen gives the skin resiliency and elasticity. The body's production of new collagen slows with aging. Vitamin C, one of the least expensive antiaging remedies, helps to build and maintain collagen and elastin.

Our skin contains antioxidants that excessive ultra-violet light can destroy. An antioxidant slows the aging of the skin. Certain vitamins are especially beneficial to the skin, hair and nails. They are:

| | |
|---|---|
| Vitamin A | Nails, skin, hair, eyes; antioxidant; promotes elasticity and smoothness. |
| Vitamin B$^2$ riboflavin | Nails, skin, hair and vision. |
| B complex, niacin | Skin. |
| B complex, biotin | Hair and skin. |
| Vitamin C | Antioxidant, photo-protectant. |
| Vitamin E | Strong healing qualities, photo-protectant. |
| Beta-carotene | Antioxidant. |

A daily multivitamin, containing the recommended daily allowance (RDA) for folate, iron and other important nutrients, is a good idea. We don't have to buy vitamins if we eat plenty of the following natural sources:

| | |
|---|---|
| Vitamin A | Milk and dairy products, yellow fruits, green and yellow vegetables, egg yolk. |
| Vitamin B | Milk and dairy products, eggs, nuts, seeds, citrus fruits, brewer's yeast, enriched cereals, green vegetables, fish, liver, lean meat. |
| Vitamin C | Fresh fruits and vegetables. |
| Vitamin E | Vegetable oils, whole raw seeds and nuts, soybeans.[2] |

Cod liver oil, an old cure and a natural source of Vitamins A and D, alleviates dryness in skin and hair, helps arthritis, strengthens bones and the immune system, and lubricates all body linings. To eliminate the fishy taste, it is processed in mint, cherry and orange flavors. Dale Alexander, recognized for his comprehensive research on the remedial powers of cod liver oil, has lectured extensively and written four books on the subject. In his book, *Dry Skin and Common Sense*,[3] he recommends using one teaspoon to one tablespoon of liquid cod liver oil (not the capsule form) mixed with four ounces of milk or orange juice. Blend with one-half a banana for potassium. For the best assimilation throughout the body, drink one hour before eating.

## *Move it!*

Just as constant flow keeps mountain streams pure, so exercise stimulates the flow of blood throughout the body and keeps it powerful. People exercise so they can live happily and harmoniously without a complaining physique. When the body is vigorously exercised, the skin gets a healthy hue and produces more collagen. Collagen plumps up facial lines. The increased oxygen intake also aids in the production of new cells. Increased circulation brings nutrients to the cells and organs and retards the aging of the skin, the largest organ of the body. Channels open and motile energy fills the body; we find capacities we did not know we had. It is no exaggeration to say that intelligent exercising is the best known anti-aging pill.

Experts believe that regular exercise reduces the causes of many diseases, increases longevity and comfort of living.[4] Any activity that moves and stimulates the body wards off heart disease, stroke, brittle and broken bones, and the pain of arthritis. It also improves sleep and relaxation, lowers cholesterol, and increases flexibility of all joints. Doing Tai Chi and/or yoga daily reduces falling by 50 percent because they coordinate and strengthen muscular activity and develop flexibility.The more we put into physical action, the more energy and renewal we get back because energy begets energy. Benefits are both physical and mental. Remembering how to exercise, how to play the game, how to use weight-lifting machines, etc., exercises the mind.

If you feel more critical or grumpy than usual, physical activity eliminates the grouchies. When the physique is exercised and properly fed, not only do the hair, nails, and skin become vitalized, but attitude improves.

Explaining why she didn't exercise, Phyllis Diller quipped she's at an age where her back goes out more than she does![5] If

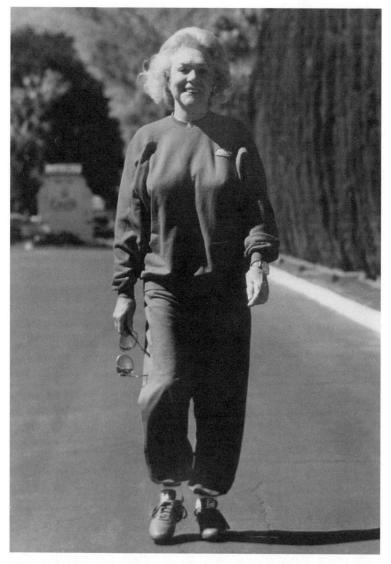

Alice Faye was a film star of the 1930s and 1940s and is wife of bandleader Phil Harris. Now in her seventies, she has been Ambassador for Good Health for Pfizer Pharmaceuticals since 1984. Her book, Growing Older, Staying Young, was published in 1990. She believes, "Once you make exercise a part of your lifestyle, you'll never want to stop ... one more tip ... for heaven's sake, have a sense of humor. It really helps you keep your spirits up."

exercise is not for you, find a suitable substitute because the advantages are too great to ignore. A gentle approach to health and rejuvenation, called Tai Chi Chih, is explained in a book by Justin F. Stone, a former Tai Chi Ch'uan teacher. The title is *Tai Chi Chih; Joy Thru Movement.* Through a series of slow, easy movements practiced daily, the body and mind are energized and cleansed.

Walking is the easiest, safest and most inexpensive. You do need good walking shoes. Strolling is okay but striding and swinging your arms is better. It is so simple. Do it anywhere. It is the best remedy for a broad spectrum of illnesses. Striding is a vital help in losing excess fat and keeping it lost.

This era of unlimited opportunities presents a variety of ways to get the body moving. Besides walking, golf, tennis, skiing, tap and line dancing, there are aquasize, swimming, fast walking, biking, hiking, yoga, weight-lifting, gentle aerobics and more. Keep the face relaxed during all physical activity to prevent tension lines. Although running has its advocates, excessive running causes facial skin to droop (skin starts to lose elasticity after 30) and other problems. Check out your community recreation and senior centers for physical activity bargains. A few dollars spent weekly will save you hundreds, even thousands in medical bills. The belief now is that if we don't take time for health activity, we will have to spend time for illness.

Ann was in a near fatal automobile accident 20 years ago that crushed both of her knees. After recuperation, she could walk without a cane, but weakness was always present and her favorite sports, tennis and ice skating, were out of the question. When she was 70, she started lifting weights under the guidance of a teacher who showed her ten steps to strengthen and tone her body. Three times a week she put on her sweats and went to the community center to "pump iron." After regularly pushing weights with her legs, she became more sure-footed than at any time since the accident. Her attitude took a happy turn, energy increased and feelings of well-being bloomed.

At the summer Senior Games in Greeley, Colorado, men and women from 55 to 80+ play tennis, swim, throw frisbees, race walk, bowl and bike race (to name only some of the events). You should see the shining faces when they win medals. Even if they weren't winners, they still pulse with a *joie de vivre,* basking in the satisfaction of team play and meeting other gutsy people over 55. The nonparticipants had to be impressed watching their peers of all shapes and ages, even two sightless swimmers, wrestling with challenges. Many train from one year to the next striving to achieve new goals.

When I asked an over-70 race walker how she maintained her slender figure, she said, "Illness, my dear, illness. I've had about everything wrong with me. Used to dive from the high board. Now I just do ordinary swimming and race walking. Sure do like the race walking. Almost won a medal, too. Maybe next year." You can believe she's training for it.

Exercise is as big a part of beauty as the facial and makeup, maybe more. The extra flush of oxygen, the pumping of the heart, the speeding up of the metabolism – all help to rejuvenate the skin and tune the body. Just as important is the mental uplift that erases depression and stress.

## Facial Massage and Exercises

Stimulating the skin by gentle massage activates the collagen fibers below the epidermis layer. Wrinkles occur when these fibers lose their flexibility. On a cleansed face, apply an emollient creme or oil. Use the fingers to gently make continuous one-inch circles over the surface of the face and throat, but not around the eye area. Try doing this in the shower or bath. The warmth of the steam causes the skin to absorb the moisture that minimizes facial lines.

Facial exercises benefit tone and texture, dilating the vascular system and bringing blood, oxygen and nutrients to the skin. Although facial exercises improve circulation, some critics claim they cause lines and wrinkles. This may happen if the face is not lubricated with a creme or oil before exercising or if it is done with jerking movements. The best movement is slow and controlled, building muscle tone and lifting sagging skin. Here are some basic how-to's:

- Cleanse, then lubricate the face. Apply an emollient with the fingers, using upward strokes or small circular motions. Be gentle.

- Squeeze and expand the muscles in the area you wish to tone and firm up. For example, on the forehead slowly raise the eyebrows high, then lower them and squint. Release slowly.

- For the eye area, first apply a moisturizing eye creme. Open eyes wide and then squeeze them tightly closed. Repeat several times.

- Devise ways to stretch and relax all areas of your face where you wish to decrease lines. Do this daily for two weeks and observe results.

- After exercising, hold a teaspoon under medium hot water until the metal is very warm. With the outside bowl of the spoon, "iron out" the lines with gentle upward strokes. As the lubricant you applied in step one penetrates the skin, think of the lines melting away.

- Blow up balloons, or blow water in your bath or shower, puffing up the skin around your mouth. This helps to keep the cheeks and "squirrel pouches" firm and tones the muscles around your lips. Spend a minute each day blowing. It also strengthens your lungs.[6]

- Head rolls are easy. Do them every day. They stimulate circulation to the entire head, eyes, face and neck, keep the throat and jaw line firm, help to control the development of a double chin and relax this whole area. With erect posture, either standing or sitting, slowly drop head down, roll to side, back (be very careful here), the other side and down to front. Do *slowly* three to five times, then roll in the other direction.[7]

## Smile!

Contrary to what some people believe, smiling does not cause wrinkles, but it can prevent them. Everything goes up! Did you ever notice how much more attractive and youthful a woman looks when she smiles? Tony Ray, a makeup artist, wrote in *The Silver/Grey Beauty Book*, "One of the best gravity-beaters is smiling! There is more to it than the mere fact that a happy face has a youthful sparkle. Smiling turns up the corners of your mouth, lifts your cheeks, and crinkles your eyes – all of which counteract the downcast look of sagging muscles."[8]

A smile is also one of our best assets, costing nothing, but saying a lot. Charm in manner and appearance is more important now than ever before. Dale Carnegie thought it was so important that he wrote an entire chapter on smiling in his classic, *How to Win Friends and Influence People*.[9] Describing a smile as "therapeutic," he recommends that even when you don't feel like smiling, do it anyway – not a forced grin but wholeheartedly. You need it, and the world needs it.

Smiling creates happiness, good will and the realization that all is not hopeless. Carnegie described a dinner party in New York City where a wealthy woman, who spent a fortune on furs, jewels and gown, was eagerly trying to make a good impression on everyone. She failed because her unsmiling face was dour and self-centered. Her expression was far more influential than her extravagant attire.

"Be cheerful. Keep the corners of your mouth turned up, and hide your worries and disappointments under a smile." – Ann Landers[10]

## *Sunscreen* _____

Dr. Thomas B. Fitzpatrick, chairman of the Department of Dermatology at Harvard Medical School, maintains his anti-aging secrets are "intellectual growth – keeping the mind active, continuing education throughout life, exercise and – perhaps most important of all, moderation in alcohol, food, tobacco, and sun exposure, all primary areas of abuse." He added, "Ninety-nine percent of premature wrinkling is caused by sun exposure."[11] Over-exposure causes loss of elasticity that results in wrinkles and lines.

As the skin matures, the epidermal cells that produce melanin, a pigment substance that protects against harmful ultraviolet rays, decrease. This changes the skin's immune response, making it more susceptible to sun damage. The skin turns pink where it used to tan.

Every day, 20 minutes before going outside, apply a sunscreen or sunblock. Slather it on if you are going to be spending long periods of time in the sun. Women are inclined to put on too little rather than too much according to dermatologist Dr. Barbara Reed. Sunscreens have sun protection factors (SPFs) from two to 50, the higher the number the greater the protection. SPF 15 is the best protection for most skin types. Very sensitive skin types should go for higher SPFs and preferably paba-free. Products are available that are chemical-free. When you expect to participate in water sports or to perspire, get one that is also waterproof. Sunscreens are available that are oil-free and that include moisturizers.

## *Puffs Under the Eyes* _____

Eye strain, stress, genetics, respiratory allergies, and too much salt in the diet are among the causes of under-eye puffiness. The skin in this area is very delicate and should be treated tenderly. Some doctors claim that regular exercise may help this condition. To reduce, do one of the following during a 15 to 20-minute relaxation period:

- Place cold compresses, such as plastic eye masks filled with cold water or cotton balls soaked in ice water, on the eye area. Or, keep two tablespoons in the refrigerator until they are cold. Hold the underside of the spoons on the puffy areas.

- Try one-half slice of cucumber or a slice from the inside an Idaho potato on each puff.

- Under each eye, place a black tea bag that has steeped for five minutes in a saucer of hot water. Lie down on a towel, press the tea bag into the skin. After 15 minutes, cleanse.

If you wake in the morning with puffiness, press a washcloth that has been dipped in cold water on the area. Cold water is a good toner. Makeup also helps. Place a white or light shade concealant in the indents under the puffiness and a foundation that is slightly darker than your regular tint on top of the puffs. Blend edges.

## Complexion Care

Correct skin care creates a youthful complexion. It pays big dividends. Skin is a sensitive organ. A simple routine is valuable to keep it healthy and lessen signs of aging. There is no guarantee that lines will disappear, but they will lessen. The more consistent you are, the better your face will look. Think of it as a preserving process, not a laborious one.

Proper skin care saves time in applying makeup because the complexion develops an even texture and cosmetics glide on. It involves five steps: cleansing, exfoliating, toning (optional), moisturizing and protecting. If you think that is too much, simplify. Do only what your skin requires.

Here are a few basic tips:

- What you do to the face, do to the throat, all around the throat.

- Use upward-moving gentle strokes when cleansing and moisturizing.

- Never roughly push or pull the facial skin.

- Use the ring finger with a gentle touch on the fragile area around the eyes.

- Never use hot water. It strips away the protective oil in the skin that retains moisture.

*Cleansing.* Daily cleansing is the secret to an ageless complexion, because it increases the skin's receptivity to moisturizing. An effective cleanser leaves the skin feeling soft and smooth, not greasy or dry. Use the correct product for your skin type and rinse thoroughly, many splashings, with warm water and a washcloth. A washcloth provides a slight abrasive that easily removes stubborn makeup and debris.

If you like a bar, look for a nonalkaline, soap-free cleansing product. It rinses easier than soap and is milder. Soaps wash away natural oils, causing dryness, and may also leave a film. A non-soap bar may be called a beauty or complexion bar without the word "soap" on the label. These products have most of the advantages and few of the disadvantages of soap.

You may think that your mother (or grandmother) used soap and water and their complexion was beautiful, so why not me? According to *The Standard Book for Professional Estheticians*,* "Your grandmother may have been one of those people who had a naturally healthy and attractive skin. However, she was not confronted with some of the enemies of the skin that have come about in recent times. Air pollution, chemicals in water, preservatives in food are just a few of the things in our modern environment that may affect the skin. Today it is more important than ever to give the skin proper, daily care."

For dry skin, massage on olive oil (it easily removes all makeup) and thoroughly rinse off with warm water. When you cleanse at night, it is unnecessary to cleanse again in the

---

* Reprinted by permission of Milady Publishing Company from *The Standard Book for Professional Estheticians* by Joel Gerson.

morning. Just rinse with cool water. Besides stimulating circulation, cool water constricts the capillaries, invigorating and firming the skin tissue.

*Steam Cleaning.* This warm watery diffusion on the face and throat

- Softens dulling dead surface cells so they are more easily removed

- Penetrates the skin, loosens deposits of grease, blackheads, makeup or dirt for a more effective cleaning

- Opens pores to eliminate toxins

- Increases blood circulation and oxygen because the blood vessels expand

- Refreshes, moisturizes and temporarily softens lines. This adds up to a healthier and improved skin tone.

Facial steam or vaporizing machines are easy to use and beautify the complexion. They are available from drug stores and beauty supply stores. As the vapor out, move your face around so that the whole surface and the throat feel the benefit.

You can also use the "pot" method: Fill a pot with one quart of water, cover, and bring to a boil. Turn off the heat, remove the cover. Place a towel over your head and the pot, creating a tent to catch the steam. Then, lean over the pot eight to 12 inches from the water. Do not put your face too close or you risk burning.

In preparation for both methods, cleanse first. Protect the delicate areas around the eyes and lips with a light creme. Be sure no emollient is on the rest of your face or throat to block the effectiveness of the mist. Close your eyes during the process. Eye pads are not necessary. Vaporizing helps the lines around the eye area. It only takes five to ten minutes once a week. Allow five minutes or less for dry, sensitive skin. Complete by rinsing with warm water. Double the benefits now – moisturize, mask or exfoliate.

*Exfoliating/Masking.* Skin cells reproduce once a month. Old ones are sloughed off. Buildup of old, dead cells gives skin a dull, scaly, uneven texture that prevents oxygen and moisture from penetrating to the live cells underneath. Consequently, lines are magnified. The skin functions better when buildup is removed by exfoliating or masking. Cleansing does not do this.

Jeffrey Bruce, a makeup artist, said in his book *About Face* (Putnam Publishing Group), "If you've never exfoliated before (shame!), now you really have no choice. Age brings an accumulation of dead skin cells which, left to their own devices, give a coarse, thick appearance. The dead surface skin must be removed if you're not to look like the alligator lady at the circus…"[12] Exfoliating and masking products contain granules that scrub away useless debris, giving the complexion a healthy shine. They do not replace the cleansing process, they improve upon it. Some also moisturize.

Select one according to your skin type – dry, normal, combination or oily. Exfoliate or mask after cleansing, twice a week for dry skin and three times for oily. For combination skin, mask a third time in oily areas only. Massage the product on your face and throat. Do not mask or exfoliate the eye area or where the skin is broken out or irritated. The best time is before retiring.

For a homemade mask, try one of the following. Leave it on for 15 to 20 minutes according to your comfort level. Rinse with warm water, then cool.

- One whipped egg white
- One-fourth cup of thick buttermilk
- One egg yolk and two tablespoons of honey mixed into a paste
- One teaspoon of plain yogurt and one teaspoon of honey, mix
- A paste of water and oatmeal

- Mix one teaspoon of baking powder with one egg white or one teaspoon of Cetaphil lotion.

*Alpha Hydroxy Acid Products (AHAs).* AHAs are also exfoliaters. These home-use lotions and cremes are a significant development in treating aging skin. "Scientific studies have shown that products containing alpha hydroxy acids, when used consistently for a period of time, can improve the appearance of dry wrinkled skin by mild peeling of the surface cells," said Linda Fang, M.D.,[13] dermatologist and developer of the Linda Sý Skin Care System. Although they do not prevent the aging of the skin, they do make it more youthful-looking. It may take four to six weeks to see a noticeable difference especially if you are using a product with a low AHA concentration of from one to eight percent.

Nontoxic alpha hydroxy acids are found in natural foods. For example:

Glycolic acid is derived from sugar cane
Lactic acid, from soured milk
Malic acid, from apples
Citric acids, from citrus fruits
Tartaric acid, from grapes, berries, passion fruit and red wine
Gluconic acid, from corn.

Lactic and glycolic acids are the most common. Experts claim glycolic acid works faster because it has the smallest molecular structure of all AHAs. It has more exfoliating properties. Lactic acid is gentler, with moisturizing properties. Both penetrate the skin. There is no evidence, however, that one works better than the other. In general, they:

- Remove dead cells from the outer layer of the skin (cleansing doesn't do this), peel away old skin, and lessen wrinkles after longtime use

- Enable the skin to absorb moisturizing better. Skin acts healthier, looks younger and is a little firmer

- Neutralize free radical damage (the aging of the skin)

- Soften lines and lighten spots, discolorations and freckles

- Unclog pores and reduce large ones; clear up blackheads and whiteheads; sometimes they help to clear blemishes

- Restore smoothness to rough, cracked, chapped or thickened skin that is dry because of arid climates or skin diseases

- Make skin radiant and less likely to show discolorations when used correctly and regularly. Clarifies the ashen look of black skin.

The percentage of AHA in a product determines its ability to exfoliate and to give you maximum benefits. The higher the percentage of AHA content, the stronger it is. An 12% to 15% AHA concentration gives noticeable results quicker. Aqua Glycolic lotion, a 12% AHA, is available over the counter from some drugstores and pharmacies. Lac Hydrin, also a 12% AHA, and those with 15% require a prescription.

Skin care centers and dermatologists sell these products. Most skin care lines have AHA cremes, lotions and gels. Good ones are available in drug and grocery stores for under $10 and you get as much for your buck, and sometimes more, as you would with the higher-priced ones in department stores.

Many cosmetic lines have AHAs for normal/dry, sensitive, and oily skin. For dry skin, get an AHA that moisturizes and is fragrance and alcohol free. A creme is more emollient than a lotion and is better for very dry skin, especially in those seasons when the skin feels dehydrated. Oily skin requires an oil-free AHA gel.

If you have sensitive skin, look for one specifically labeled for this type such as *Alpha Hydrox's Sensitive Skin, Pond's Age Defying Creme for Sensitive Skin,* or one with low AHA content.

Read the directions and follow religiously. Apply to a cleansed face. Do not use soap or any cleanser that leaves a film that can neutralize or prevent penetration. For this reason, many cosmetic companies have their own cleansers. Smooth a pea-size amount on your entire face. Apply it immediately after bathing when skin is damp to boost moisture retention. Use sparingly around the lips and eyes. Any tingling sensation should diminish. You can start by using it every other night, gradually increasing to every night. When you apply it before retiring, lightly rinse your face in the morning to remove any flaking that may appear then moisturize. Or, you can apply the AHA during the day, wait for it to penetrate, then put on make-up. Otherwise, the ingredients in the foundation will neutralize the AHA.

Do not slather it on, thinking you will get quicker results! Overdosing can cause irritation. Women sometimes do this and their skin begins to flake. If your skin starts to flake and itch, stop using for a few days and/or go to a lower concentration. Continual use is necessary if you want to keep the benefits. Stop and the skin goes back to its original condition. Keep the AHA (sunscreen, all products) out of the eyes.

Although the directions may suggest application twice a day, keep in mind the alpha hydroxy acid is an irritant and thins the skin. Once a day or every other day may be sufficient if the percentage of AHA is over 10%. Monitor your skin. If there is no redness or flaking, your application is correct. A sunscreen with SPF 15 is recommended.

*Other uses of alpha hydroxy acid products.* The facial AHA product can be used on the throat and hands. You don't need two, one for face and another for the body and hands. Massage a non-alcohol, 8% or more AHA creme or lotion into cuticles to remove dry rough skin. Women of color can use an AHA combined with hydroquinone (a bleaching agent) to lighten dark spots caused by breakouts. This combination also bleaches age spots on the back of hands. AHA shampoos help to exfoliate accumulated dead cells that linger on the scalp. *Alpha Hydrox* has 4%, 10% and 12% foot cremes that moisturize and exfoliate dry rough skin.

*Toning (Optional).* Apply a toner with a cotton ball. Moisten if skin is very sensitive and avoid the eye and lip areas.

This step restores the protective acid balance and seems to "wake up" the skin. Use an astringent like witch hazel for oily areas to absorb excess oil.

> Large pores? Mix one egg yolk and same amount of plain yogurt. Let dry on your face for a half hour. Wash off.

*Moisturizing.* Moisturizers are lifesavers for dry complexions and the answer to a healthy, glowing, comfortable face. Some contain a sunscreen and a tint. They lubricate, soften fine lines and reduce flaking. Because they hydrate the membrane, the skin has a dewier, younger look. Apply to damp skin because it absorbs better than dry. Put on your foundation after it is absorbed.

> Night-time nourishment for the face: Dab on a pure, unperfumed oil – avocado, olive, vitamin E – on driest spots. Smooth in with wet fingers.

*A wise word of caution.* Do not use heavy cremes or oils around the eyes. When they seep in, the result is blurred vision.

*Protection.* Foundation protects the skin from dehydrating conditions, environmental pollutants and, to a degree, harmful sun rays. Some foundations contain sunscreen and moisturizers. When you use separate products, the order of application is sunscreen, moisturizer, foundation.

## Rosacea (pronounced rose-ay-shah)

Rosacea is a chronic facial condition that causes redness, pimples, red lines and nasal bumps. Remember W.C. Fields with his big, red nose? That was his problem. Rosacea can be controlled, but as of this date, it cannot be cured. Early treatment prevents it from getting worse. About 70 percent to 80 percent of rosacea patients notice significant improvement with prescribed oral or topical medications or a combination of both.

Avoid skin care products or cosmetics that contain alcohol (check hair spray, too), witch hazel, fragrance, acetone, menthol, peppermint, eucalyptus oil, clove oil, salicylic acid, oil, graininess, or irritants. Apply a dermatologist-recommended moisturizer as needed after the medication has dried. Whenever you think you will be in the sun use an SPF 15 or higher sunscreen.

In addition to medical therapy, rosacea can be controlled by proper cleansing.

- Wash your face twice a day, morning and evening. Be sure to remove all makeup at night. Use a gentle cleanser, such as Cetaphil, Ponds Foaming Face Wash, or Dove, and apply with a soft shaving brush or natural sponge.

- Remove the cleanser by splashing several times with tepid or cool water, or use a sheet of sterilized cotton. Dry flaky skin is soothed by following up with Metro Cream (Galderma Laboratories).

- Do not use toners or astringents. They may irritate or inflame the skin.

- Let your face dry 30 minutes before applying topical medication or makeup. Makeup effectively camouflages rosacea. Use oil-free, fragrance-free cosmetics that list water first in the list of ingredients. Use a color-correcting prefoundation base in sheer green to counter redness.

The pulse dye laser, used by dermatologists and cosmetic surgeons, eliminates the redness from rosacea. Once the redness is reduced, the breakouts decrease or disappear altogether. After laser treatment the skin appears darkened but this disappears in 10 to 14 days. More about laser surgery is found on page 91.

The National Rosacea Society, 220 South Cook Street, Suite 201, Barrington, Illinois 60010, publishes a newsletter, *Rosacea Review.* It reports success stories in the fight against rosacea, the latest advances in treatments, a QA column that invites your questions, seasonal tips, and other helpful information.

## *How to Select Skin Savers*

1. Ask about returning the product if you have an adverse reaction or find it doesn't do what the advertising claims.

2. Quality products are available at economical prices.

3. Always read the directions.

4. For dry or sensitive skin, look for products that are allergy-free, no alcohol or fragrance. The words unscented and fragrance-free are used interchangeably. Some products marked as unscented or fragrance-free may still have traces of scent to dull the chemical smell of the ingredients. Look for the words "100% fragrance free."

5. Select products for your skin type:

   *Dry to normal skin* has small pores with little or no secretion apparent. Products for dry skin restore the skin's optimum moisture balance. Products for normal skin preserve its balance of oil and moisture and give mature skin a healthy texture.

   *Combination skin* may be dry, but oil appears on the T-zone (center of forehead, nose and mouth). Products for combination skin control excess oil in the T-zone. They leave dry areas moist and supple and restore the skin's moisture balance.

   *Oily skin* has frequent secretion and large pores. Oil-free products help to control oiliness.

   Wherever you have an occasional breakout, use oil-free products.

6. Look for the following words that are frequently used in products and in advertisements:

Collagen – A protein that binds moisture to the skin and gives the skin firmness and elasticity.

Elastin – A protein substance in the skin that gives it firmness and elasticity. Products with collagen and elastin help to control the aging process.

Dimethicone – An emollient that helps to condition and protect the skin.

Dehydrates – Removes moisture from skin.

Hydrates – Adds moisture.

Rehydrates – Restores normal moisture balance.

Emollient – A lubricant that is soothing, softening, and may retard fine lines. Creams have the most emollients.

Exfoliant – An ingredient or product (such as a grainy cream) used to remove the outermost layer of dead cells.

Humectant – An ingredient such as collagen that helps the skin to retain moisture.

Hypoallergenic or allergy-free – Screened to eliminate all known irritants.

Non-comedogenic – Does not clog pores, or cause blackheads, whiteheads, blemishes.

Occlusive – Seals in moisture.

Stearic acid – A lubricant that relieves dryness by helping to reduce moisture loss.

Syndet – A synthetic detergent; a non-alkaline, soap-free cleansing product. It is mild, gentle and rinsable.

7. Natural Organic Products. More companies are using plants to produce cremes, lotions, sun blocks and makeup. This does not automatically make the products better for

the skin. Eucalyptus, camphor, thyme, lavender, peppermint and cornstarch are irritants and can cause allergic
reactions. Ginseng, horsetail, tea tree oil, aloe vera, apricot
oil, calendula and evening primrose oil are beneficial.
Major cosmetic lines use some plant-based ingredients
in their products. Others, the so-called "green" beauty
companies are based on organics. You will find these in
natural food stores and some supermarkets.

8.  Ingredients are listed on the product or the box according to
    amount with the highest quantity first and the lowest, last.
    For example, when a product is advertised as having vita-
    min E or collagen, notice its location in the ingredient list to
    find out how much is in the product. *A Consumer'
    Dictionary of Cosmetic Ingredients* by Ruth Winter defines
    chemical and plant names to help you identify those that
    are good and bad.

9.  Cellular renewal and nutritional ingredients rejuvenate the
    appearance of mature skin. Some of these are: vitamins A
    and E, panthenol (a vitamin B complex factor), lecithin,
    shea butter (karite butter), hyaluronic acid, sodium PCA
    (NaPCA), linoleic acid, shark liver oil, aloe vera extract,
    jojoba oil, avocado oil, wheat germ oil, gotu kola extract.

10. Skin rejuvenators are gels or creams manufactured by
    leading cosmetic companies and many smaller ones. Their
    formulations help aging skin. In general, they:

    - Temporarily minimize fine lines by tightening and
      firming the skin and reducing puffiness
    - Improve suppleness by moisturizing within the
      epidermis
    - Work under the skin to reduce lines
    - Restore a youthful glow
    - Shield from sun damage with paba-free protection.

Centuries ago women ground powders and mixed com-
pounds, concocting creams, oils and mud packs to preserve
their skin, or they sadly accepted as inevitable the aging look.

With today's scientific advances, we have products that are easy to use, lightweight, and non-irritating. Safe products are abundant with even better ones to come.

*Kitchen Aids.* If you forgot to buy a skin care product or want to save money, here are some suggestions. Gently massage them on face and throat.

Cleansing – Any cold-pressed oil. Olive and safflower are good choices. Or, two to three tablespoons of plain yogurt. Apply to damp skin. Rinse thoroughly.

Exfoliating – Make a paste with yellow cornmeal and water. Rinse with warm water followed by a cool splash.

Toning – One-half teaspoon apple cider vinegar into eight ounces of water.

Nourishing – One of the following: a thin layer of the margarine sold in health food stores that contains no artificial colorings, flavorings or preservatives; a light application of mayonnaise; a light application of olive or any cold-pressed oil.

Without reliable information on kitchen ingredients, you could end up using some that clog the pores, or that are too oily or too drying for your skin.

## Product Workability

The claims made by cosmetic manufacturers are the results of years of research and hundreds of tests. This means that in the majority of tests, the reactions were as advertised. It may or may not work for you. Each person's body chemistry is different. It reacts uniquely to foods and topical treatments. When a product does not work as advertised, the reasons are it is inappropriate for your body chemistry, you are using it incorrectly, the product is not what it claims to be, or it is defective.

When purchasing a product from a knowledgeable salesperson, ask questions until you are satisfied about proper use, what it will do and if you can return an unsatisfactory item.

Reputable companies, conscious of the competition in the marketplace, want customers to be happy with their merchandise and willingly make an adjustment for good will.

---

The expensive complexes for reducing lines and wrinkles do not replace or eliminate the necessity of THE BIG FOUR: healthy eating habits, drinking plenty of water, planned physical activity (as defined in "Why Exercise?"), and a daily cleansing routine. They are the eternal prescriptions for beauty and well-being.

## Body Skin Care

Although the skin care steps for the body are the same as for the face, the ingredients in the products may differ because the skin on the face is more delicate than the rest of the body. Body buffing creams perform the same function as the facial mask, or you can rub away dead surface cells with a soft body brush or loofah, then bathe.

Since water is very important, hydrate for 10 to 20 minutes by relaxing in a bathtub with one of these:

- a bath gel
- a natural oil
- half a cup of powdered milk
- the oil from two vitamin E capsules
- one cup of baking soda.

Add a couple drops of your favorite fragrance. While soaking, read a book, listen to music or the radio, snack, eat a juicy orange, sip your favorite drink, or just let your mind and body drift. Let the water seep in. This is your personal time.

Pat dry, leaving the skin moist and, if you didn't use a bath oil, apply a moisturizer for silky smoothness. With the warmth of the bath, the lotion will sink into the pores soothing dryness.

## *Fragrance for Loveliness*

Perfumery began as an industry about 4,000 years ago when human development expanded from the agricultural to urban life. Throughout millennia, scents and incense were used in temples for their mystifying influence in religious and devotional ceremonies. Unusual, striking scents were valuable components in healing oils and the glamour of allurement. Vials of perfume were buried in the tombs of Tutankhamen, Ramses and other Egyptian kings and queens for their convenience and use in the hereafter.

Marc Antony's fate was sealed before he even met Cleopatra. The enchantress was clothed in a flowing, diaphanous gown, cruising down the Nile in a vessel with perfumed sails. Incense wafted in the breezes surrounding her throne and her body breathed the most exotic scents. What man could resist her?

Fragrances are the ultimate body language. They delight and haunt the mind, relax and soothe, evoke moods, and create a sense of well-being. Some are relaxing to the point of diffusing stress. This sensory perception acts like a time machine, conjuring up memories of people and places.

Referred to as bottled magic, scents add a lovely aura to femininity, subtly expressing your distinctive charm and dignity, who you are and what you are like. Because they capture the olfactory sense with a particular message, you need to select them to match your personality. Sometimes, scent is as much a part of our identity as fingerprints. Pick it to fit your moods. For the flirty and feminine, sniff out the florals. For glamour and glitz, go for an oriental or spicy scent. For just plain fun, check out the upbeat, modern fragrances. Selecting an aroma is very personal. Make it an adventure, not a hurried affair.

A unique way to decide upon a perfume, eau de toilette or cologne (listed according to potency) is spritz a little on the wrist and taste it. If reasonably pleasant to the palate, it will blend with body chemistry.

Usually, eau de toilette lasts four to six hours and reaches ten to fifteen feet. In some old-line French fragrances, the eau de toilette is weaker than the cologne. If the price doesn't show this, the salesperson should know. Cologne lasts one to four hours and reaches two to eight feet. Alcohol-based fragrances (cologne, eau de parfum or toilette) drop off sharply, then remain constant. Oil or cream-based scents (body lotion or bath oil worn as cologne) taper off gradually. Herbal oil fragrances, with citrus and floral bouquets, have good aromatic quality and come in small bottles, easy to carry in the purse. When heavy fragrances no longer seem appropriate, sniff around men's colognes that have a cleaner, fresher scent.

Fragrance fade-out is a frequent problem especially for dry skin. Solve this by

- Using oriental, musk, or heady floral scents rather than citrus.

- Applying a moisturizer first, then the fragrance. The oils in the lotion help to "hold" the fragrance.

- Trying an oil based formula, such as a body lotion, bath or herbal oil. Touch up with perfume or cologne.

Wear it on the pulse points: behind ears, on the inside wrists and elbows, at the base of the throat or even behind the knees. For lasting power, layer by using talc, cologne or eau de toilette and finishing with perfume. Why not combine scents? If your skin is allergic to fragrance, saturate a cotton ball and tuck in your clothing where it will not irritate the skin, or use an herbal oil fragrance.

When going to bed, even if you are alone, smooth on a scented body lotion, dust with scented powder, or put fragrance on pillow case, sheet or nightie. Why? Because anything that gives a sense of loveliness is good for the psyche. Pamper yourself with the luxurious feeling of a tranquil aromatic. Marilyn Monroe said she wore Chanel No. 5 to bed and that was about all.

# 3

# Be Your Own Makeup Artist

Before my makeup classes, I always ask the women why they want to learn about makeup. One woman said, "I'm 81 and think there's so much ugliness in the world that I want to see what can be done about me." During the class we saw how cosmetics took years off her face and beautified all the women present. When we finished, there were smiles all around the table.

For centuries women have been fascinated with cosmetics because they are tools for opening the door of opportunity. As mood-altering agents, they change the way we feel about our face, body and even our abilities. They enhance our good features and hide flaws; make us prettier; give a psychological uplift; and enable us to feel happier and more secure with our appearance. We wear makeup because it boosts self-acceptance and self-confidence.

The cosmetic industry anticipates the current and future requirements of women and develops products whose benefits are physiological and aesthetic.

Jeffrey Bruce, a well-known makeup artist, said in his book, "There is nothing more gorgeous, more appealing, than a ripened woman who has grown accustomed to her face. She isn't trying to compete with starlets when she skillfully brings out the seasoned sensuality she's earned. And the way she does that is with more, not less, makeup – more artfully applied. Because she's fighting gravity and loss of moisture, she has to compensate with better products – and she can't skimp on coverage...You simply cannot get away with a dab of blush anymore...I know too many women who spend a fortune on a new pair of boots or a great coat and then walk around with the same, tired face, because they've been brainwashed to believe that makeup should be drastically reduced after forty."[2]

## The Inner Artist

Every woman has an intuitive artistic sense. Look at a woman's appearance or home, and you will see how active the inner artist is in her life. Some women fully express this intuitive perception in the home, garden, handiwork or the arts, but when it comes to their appearance, they turn it off.

The inner artist frequently manifests during makeup classes with the placement of colorings. During the discussion of blush, I applied it to Lucy's face and asked her how she liked it. She replied, "It's fine, but I would like it a little closer to my nose." So we blended the color over a degree, and the class agreed they liked it better, too. Although Lucy knew little about makeup techniques, she analyzed, listened to her intuition, and the other women agreed that it was an improvement.

Boredom never sets in when we listen to our inner artist for variety in application and color selection. The more we listen to this intuitive artistic sense, the more confidence we have in our face and fashion potential. When this sense is fully actualized, no expert can improve upon its ideas for your beauty.

## Key Points

Most women know very little about applying makeup. Mary said she went to a department store cosmetic counter to get a little education. The all-knowing salesperson proceeded to apply intense colors without asking her what she liked or preferred. Embarrassed by the vivid shades, which she noticed were similar to what the salesperson was wearing, Mary rushed home, hoping no one she knew would see her. This is a fairly common experience. In fact, one woman said she was so intimidated by department store clerks that she had a beauty consultant who came to her home and gave her honest opinions.

As you venture into the world of cosmetic artistry, consider the following guidelines:

1   Organize your cosmetics and applicators. Throw out old makeup. Today's products are far superior in content and color.

2.  Before you go shopping, think through what you want so you won't be talked into buying something you won't use. Talk to the representative whose face you admire, one over 50 if possible. Test the products and stay in control! Buy only what *you* like, not what he/she likes.

3.  If you have noticeable lines or wrinkles, buy matte, no-shine cosmetics – no oily-looking foundation or blush, iridescent eye shadow or metallic lip colors. Shine accentuates lines and wrinkles.

4.  Look for muted shades unless you are dark-complected. If the colors are intense-looking in the package, use a light touch when applying. Practice on the back of your hand.

5.  Whether you are a beginner or advanced in makeup application, put it on slowly and thoughtfully. If you are pinched for time, put on less but do it right. Whenever makeup is sloppy, it looks wrong. When your hand needs steadying, sit and place your elbow on the table.

6.  Practice the techniques, adapt them to your preference, be creative and have fun. If you make a mistake, so what? Redo until you like it.

7.  When you have finished, check your face by daylight or its equivalent to see that the shades beautify and are of suitable intensity. When all shades are in balance, no color, such as

eye shadow or lip color, shouts over another. **The purpose of makeup is to bring out the beauty of the woman, not the makeup.**

8.  Because you need daylight, or quality light for application, you may wish to have your makeup and mirror in a location that has indirect natural light, maybe a dressing table by a window. If this is not possible, find a makeup mirror with lighting controls and use the daylight or home light setting. Lighted makeup mirrors are inexpensive and available at discount stores.

9.  If it's difficult to see without your glasses, purchase inexpensive magnifying glasses from drug stores or mail order houses. The lenses move up and down on hinges so that you can move one lens down while seeing through the other. Or, get a double, triple or quintuple magnified mirror.

Speaking of mirrors, let's stop being intimidated by them! When you get up in the morning and look at the bland face staring back at you, remember you can transform it. Makeup artist Jeffrey Bruce said he saw Sophia Loren without her makeup and "believe me, she doesn't look so hot."[3] Few women over 50 look as good without makeup as they do with it. Thinking positively about the image we have is reinforcing mental homework, not egotism or pollyannaism. In this era of miracles, I think what makeup does for our faces is one of them. When you put energy and persistence into creating a lovely face and thinking positive about yourself, the lines and wrinkles will become insignificant. Ideas for improvement will surface. I have seen this hundreds of time in my makeup classes.

## Tools

Your fingers are often the best tools for blending everything, even eye shadow.

*100% Cotton Balls or Pads.* One hundred percent cotton has no abrasives. Anything abrasive, such as tissues that contain wood fibers, can upset sensitive skin. Cotton balls and pads are used to apply freshener, blend powder blush, remove excess makeup, or dab powder to lips to give the color more staying power.

*Cotton, Cosmetic, and Sponge Tips.* Cosmetic cotton tips are not as fuzzy as the regular cotton ones. These may be used for blending eye shadow, removing excess eye makeup, and blending corrective and tinting foundation. Use them to

- Soften edges of eye shadow so there are no unnatural lines,
- Edge a line of shadow under lower lashes,
- Erase smudges; dip first in moisturizer, if you wish,
- Touch up the lip line after applying color,
- Cover blemishes; dip in foundation and dab.

Blend a concealer under eyes where there are dark areas. Sponge tips are excellent to blend eye shadow. Wash sponge tips frequently to maintain cleanliness and purity of color.

*Sponges.* Damp-dry sponges are useful for an even application of foundation. The edges of triangular sponges may get makeup into corners and creases and may be used the same as cotton tips.

*Brushes.* Brushes come in different sizes for the application of blush, loose powder, lip color, eye shadow and the brows. They are fun to work with. Use the size that is easiest for you. As with sponges, clean regularly with soap and water. You may wish to soak them in alcohol periodically for sanitary reasons. Cleanliness is important because it's possible for bacterial buildup to cause irritation to the skin that you may incorrectly attribute to a product.

*Blotters.* They are available in 100-percent linen and are helpful in blotting oily areas during the day without disturbing makeup.

*The Organizer.* To carry cosmetics in your handbag, a plastic bag with a locking top or zipper saves the frustration of digging around to find what you want. It weighs almost nothing and you can see the contents at a glance.

## Foundation for the Natural Look _____

Foundation is as important to your face as seams are to a dress. Also called makeup or base, it is indispensable if you want your makeup to look like it comes from the inside to the outside. Foundation creates a patina that gives blended softness to the other colorings. Some contain a moisturizer and sunscreen.

Tinting foundation conceals minor imperfections. It evens out irregular pigmentation, covers pores and protects the complexion from dehydration, city pollution and ultraviolet rays, especially if it has a sun protection factor. The fifty-plus woman wants a quality foundation (she may have to pay more for this than any other makeup), one specifically for mature skin that covers well. More leading cosmetic companies are producing this type of foundation with a large selection of colors.

Finding the right shade is often difficult. This was illustrated during a makeup class. As Madeline was putting on foundation, the rest of us could not help watching because it was turning her face a mummy-like grey. When we mentioned it, she groaned and said with exasperation, "I have two bottles of foundation at home that I don't like, and I just bought this today. I never seem to get the right shade." It was even more shocking when she put on lip color because it matched the foundation!

We removed everything and started over with warmer shades. These flattering tints revitalized her face and brought out her expressive eyes; the wrong shades neutralized them. The problem was the undertones of her skin were yellow while those of the foundation and lipstick she purchased were bluish. Madeline liked muted colors, but when this foundation with cool tones interacted with her golden undertones, the result was disastrous. She wanted softer shades and these are just as available in the warm colors as they are in the cool ones.

**Selecting the Correct Shade.** Some cosmetic companies color code their foundations according to warm, cool or neutral.

Choose two or three shades that appeal to you. Place them on an area with no makeup – on the jawline or wrist where you can see it. See how they blend with your skin. One will practically disappear while others look like blobs. The shade that blends with your skin is the right one.

Foundation should match the skin on the throat. Too light a shade makes the complexion pasty-looking, too dark emphasizes lines and wrinkles. You want one that enriches your face. Some women with very fair complexions are uncomfortable with a foundation that matches the throat. They think the light shade makes their face look colorless and older. A slightly darker foundation gives a more youthful tone. Care should be taken to get the "un-madeup" look. Avoid a difference between the color of the foundation and the throat by fading out the edges at the sides of the face and under the jawbone.

*Creme or Liquid.* Creme foundation (often in a compact) is oil-based and fights dryness, giving a slight sheen, extra lubrication, heavier coverage and protection from dehydration. Powder/creme foundation provides a matte finish and good coverage.

The liquid or water-based foundation can be used by all skin types and has a matte finish, unless it contains a moisturizer. A moisturing agent creates sheen. For some complexions this is youthful. Coverage is sheerer than the creme foundation.

Oily and/or acne-prone skin requires a foundation that is 100 percent oil-free. This product has absorbing ingredients that reduce oil breakthrough and it stays fresher longer.

> A light shade of foundation
> makes a face look wider. A darker one
> makes it look narrower.

For the added protection of a sunscreen or if your skin is dry, get a foundation that is labeled accordingly. If you wish to apply your own, the order of application is: (1) moisturizer,

(2) sunscreen, (3) foundation. Allow whatever you put on your face before foundation to completely penetrate your skin. If you don't, it will absorb the foundation and dilute the color.

*Application.* Pat liquid foundation around the face with your fingers or a damp-dry sponge. Blend color with downward strokes. This stroke covers pores better. Never push or pull the skin. Glide over the surface into every nook and cranny. Do it *slowly* so that coverage is even, with no patches of too much or too little color. For the nonshiny base dust *lightly* with translucent powder.

> The extra time spent to apply foundation
> carefully is the base for a
> natural-looking, professional finish.

## Concealers/Concealants

Concealers come in different colors and have been around since the 1950s when Max Factor marketed Erace. Today's brands moisturize and have SPFs. Although some are advertised as long-wearing, the most durable are waterproof. They have many uses, such as

- Filling in tiny lines;
- Lightening dark areas;
- Covering spots, broken blood vessels, birthmarks and some scars;
- Toning down pink or ruddy pigmentation and lightening bluish areas around the eyes;
- "Bringing out" depressions and "receding" fleshiness.

One student said she was always embarrassed because her throat was red and sometimes people commented on it. When she applied a concealer to this area, she was amazed at the way it neutralized the reddish tone. On another woman, a large brown spot on her cheek magically disappeared when she covered it with a concealer and then her regular foundation.

Pigmentation problems, such as scars and birthmarks, are more effectively covered by cosmetic correctives such as Dermablend and Covermark. They are specifically formulated for this purpose. They also hide varicose veins.

## Contouring

Light shades bring out; dark ones recede. That is the basic rule of contouring.

This technique gives the illusion of more or less shape. By carefully blending the edges of the contour color, the effect is subtle, and the technique invisible. Foundation, concealers, creme or powder blush, even eye shadow offer the possibility of contouring.

Analyze your face and identify the place you want to redesign.

- If your cheeks are fleshy, place a darker shade below the cheekbones and fade out toward the jawbone with a lighter shade on the upper part of the cheekbones.

- To widen a narrow face, apply blush horizontally along the line of the cheekbones and toward the ears.

- To "narrow" a broad nose, blend a slightly darker shade of foundation on the sides.

- "Shorten" a long nose by blending a darker foundation around the tip and under the nose.

- "Lengthen" a short nose by blending a light or white shade down the middle, carefully fade it into the foundation on the sides.

- For a broad forehead or face, place a darker foundation on sides of the forehead and face. Blend into your regular foundation.

- For depressions at the temples, hollow cheeks or indents around under-eye bags, use a very light shade.

## *The Magic of Makeup*

Think of yourself as an artist and your face as the canvas. You're going to create a masterpiece! Don't laugh. You may be pleasantly surprised. During a Glamour for Grandmas class, I asked who wanted to try eye shadow. A woman with creamy white hair said, "Well, I would." Her eyes were sky blue. She was wearing a matching shirt, so I blended a pastel on the eye lids, fading it up to the brows, defined her brows with a blond pencil, tinted her cheeks with blush and applied pale pink to her lips. I couldn't stop with the shadow because the change was getting better and better. The "ohs" and "ahs" came from everyone. "You look so much younger!" someone exclaimed and others agreed. I went back to my chair. Looking at her from across the table, I was amazed at the way makeup had brightened her hair. It glowed! That's how color reacts with color. The right facial colorings enliven the face *and* the hair.

Do your makeup after deciding what you're going to wear. Coordinate colors of your makeup and clothing. An office manager I worked with wore a plum lip color and blush every day of the week and month, regardless of whether her clothing was blue, black, red or pink. Her face got boring and her makeup frequently clashed with her clothing. Someone probably told her the plum colors were her best colors. Probably they were with the outfit she was wearing at the time, but not with everything in her closet and not every day!

If you have only one lip color and one blush, it's time to emancipate your glamour box. Using a variety of shades is part of the fun and offers you flexibility to be more creative. Re-assess your makeup periodically. Julie Davis said, "New makeup techniques lose their value if the cosmetics you apply aren't up to snuff....If the color is wrong, murky oxblood lipstick instead of clear red, you won't look as great as you could. Many women will keep using the wrong cosmetics out of force of habit. Take time to evaluate your collection."[4]

Luscious shades pour into the market at the beginning of each season. When in doubt about which shade to choose, try them on your hand or place them against the apparel you want to match.

> The optimal understated makeup look is
> achieved by wearing more artfully
> applied makeup, not less.

## Eyes

People like to see eyes. We read a person through their eyes. They help us to communicate and to understand. When I ask women what they specifically want to learn about makeup, the majority say eye shadow or something involving the eyes.

The diagram shown in Illustration 1 will help you to identify the parts of the eye we describe in applying makeup.

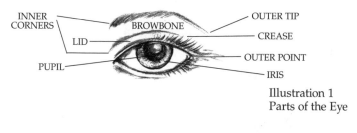

Illustration 1
Parts of the Eye

## Brows

Just as a good frame sets off a picture, sculptured brows set off the eyes. Because brows accessorize the eyes, they should be neither insignificant nor overpowering.

Frequently, change is difficult. In one class, a woman with black and white hair had white brows. When we darkened the brows to harmonize with her hair, everyone thought it looked better than the white brows and definitely more youthful. But not her! She was shocked. She had seen white brows for many years and could not accept a change now. Receptivity to change is important if you want the ageless look.

To find the natural brow line, hold a pencil diagonally from the outer edge of the nose to the outer corner of the eye. The place where the pencil touches the brow bone is the outer point. The inner point is directly over the inner corner of the eye. The natural brow line extends along the brow bone between these two points (see Illustration 2).

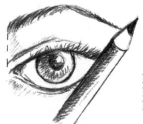

Illustration 2
Defining the Outer
Point of the Brow

The "normal" distance between the eyes equals the width of one eye (see Illustration 3). If the brows are farther from or closer to the nose than "normal" added color balances. This is described in the section *Adding Dimension to Special Eye Shapes* on page 61. The highest point on the brows is over the outer rim of the pupil.

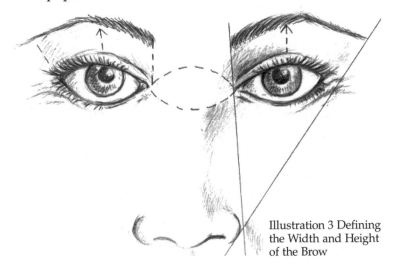

Illustration 3 Defining
the Width and Height
of the Brow

Remove stray hairs around the brows to open the area, especially when the space between the lids and brows is short.

*Sculpturing with Color.* Colorless brows are aging. Color that relates to shades in your hair, as it is now or was, is best. With white or gray hair, use taupe, blonde or slate. The brow pencil and brush-on brow powder are easy to use. The twist-up brow pencil requires no sharpening. Brush-on powder gives a soft texture. You can also mix colors, for example blond with brown, or brown with charcoal.

Thin brows are severe lines that give unnecessary sharpness. They were glamorous on Jean Harlow, but they do nothing for us. With short strokes, add color to make them fuller. The fuller brows add balance to the facial features and are gentler on lines and wrinkles.

Bushy brows are unfeminine. Brush them up, trim the excess, then brush to the side to see if they are even.

For unruly brows, put hair spray, mousse, or an emollient creme on a tooth brush and stroke the brows before going to bed and again first thing in the morning. Mousse holds best. Brow control products are also available.

Brows that are straight across without an arch "shorten" a long face.

Arched brows lengthen a round face. Do not arch too much or they take on a surprised look.

Brows that are sparse or too light in color age the face. Darken them. Start with fullness at the inner points and taper the color to the outer points. Exception: Some faces, such as the long, narrow or rectangular, require the brows to be as full at the outer points as they are at the inner points. Finish by brushing them in the same direction the hair grows.

Do not let the inner corners of the brows "hook" under. This is a downward line you do not need. Get the youthful line by adding color over the inner corners, closely paralleling the high point of the arch (see Illustration 4).

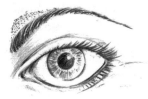

Illustration 4
Correcting the Drooping Inner Brow

The curve of the brows alters the expression of the face (see Illustration 5).

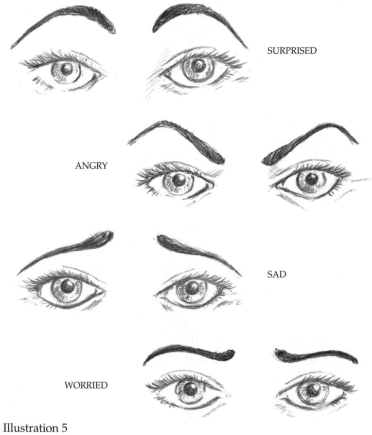

SURPRISED

ANGRY

SAD

WORRIED

Illustration 5

*No Brows.* In one of my classes, a woman said every hair on her body left after her last pregnancy three decades before. She wore an auburn wig that was perfect with her skin coloring. But with no lashes and brows, her eyes had a staring look she didn't like. With a blond brow pencil we "drew" her brows one-quarter of an inch thick at the inner corner decreasing in width to the outer tip. Along her upper and lower lashes we added eye shadow that matched the brows. She was amazed at the natural definition this gave her face and how easy it was to do.

## *Eye Shadow*

Shadow adds subtle contour. It should not scream for attention. We have all seen women with shadow that is so bright we wonder how they can look at their faces in the mirror and go out the door! SUBTLE is the magic word. Shadows come in pressed powders, cremes, pencils and watercolors. Pressed powders are easy to use. Watercolors take longer. Creme shadows tend to separate into the lines. Applying an eye lid primer or liquid foundation helps to prevent this. Matte is always best, always fashionable. Shine draws attention to lines.

When using two or three colors, blend where they meet – no endings. Sometimes we see color from the upper lash line to the crease where it stops. For the more natural look, blend it beyond the crease, fading it out gradually to the brows.

### *Placement Tips*

Keep the intense shade along the lash line. Use a pale color to lighten skin tones or shadowy places.

If you have little contour to your lids, blend a darker shade midway between the upper lid and brow. Fade it up toward the brow line.

For uplifting, parenthetical shading, blend color from the center of the lids to the outer eye corners and up to the outer points of the brows (see Illustration 6).

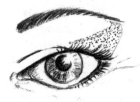

Illustration 6
Uplifting Shadow

If the space between the eye and brow is wide, apply an earth-tone foundation or beige/brown eye shadow from the crease to the brow, making the area appear narrower.

If the space between the eye and brow is narrow, apply a pale shadow from crease to the brow, making the area appear wider.

For a tinge of color place blush on the brow bone.

***Guidelines for Selecting Eye Shadow Colors.*** Shadow colors outnumber all other cosmetic colors because the jewel tones of the iris are accentuated by a wide spectrum of hues. Select colors to harmonize with your skin tone and sometimes, but not necessarily always, your outfit.

Choosing the same color as your eyes dulls the iris.

Brown shadow flatters most skin tones. Avoid blue or purple if they accentuate under-eye veins.

Aqua or lavender is good for almost everyone and plays down yellow undertones.

Light colors, such as pale pink and peach, make eyes appear larger, more open. Dark colors close them in and accent lines.

| If your irises are: | Select: |
|---|---|
| Brown | Brown, peach, green, navy |
| Brown/black | Taupe, mauve, dark green, charcoal, navy |
| Blue | Grey, sand, navy, beige, dark green |
| Green | Camel, turquoise, brown, ivory |
| Hazel | Camel, brown, green |
| Violet | Taupe, olive, mauve, dark green |

At cosmetics counters, try the shades on the back of your hand or inner wrist.

> Blue, green, or purple eye shadows
> require skillful blending to be effective.

## Lashes

Lashes with color and curl look longer. Beauty salons dye lashes with color that lasts eight to ten weeks. Use lash-thickening mascara if lashes are light in color or sparse.

Mascara thickens, conditions and adds color. Pumping the wand up and down sucks air into the tube, drying out the product. Just swirl the wand around, then remove. Bacteria easily builds up in the tube and can cause infection. Therefore, consider replacing it every three to six months to eliminate any possibility of infection. Reactions are not common, but why risk it? If your mascara stings, try the hypoallergenic brands.

*Applying Mascara.* Stroke on from roots to tips. To catch the tips, hold the wand vertical to the upper lashes and brush across, then straighten from roots to tips. For the lower lashes, hold the wand horizontal, brush across tips, then straighten (see Illustration 7).

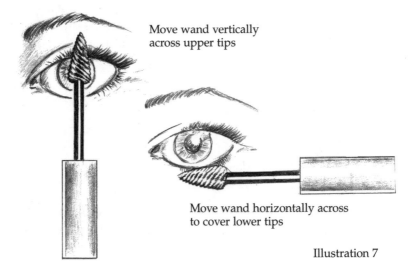

Move wand vertically
across upper tips

Move wand horizontally across
to cover lower tips

Illustration 7

Thick clumped mascara looks like thick clumped mascara. Remove clumping by separating the lashes. Use a lash comb, a small brush, or an old, clean mascara wand. To protect against flaking below the eyes, blot lashes with a tissue.

Lash curlers are popular, and so is the spoon method of crimping the lashes. Here is how it works:

1. Hold a teaspoon under hot water till warm and dry off.
2. Place the spoon in your hand with the thumb inside the concave bowl.
3. Hold the spoon so lashes are between thumb and concave bowl.
4. Press and curl up as if you were curling a ribbon.

One side takes more maneuvering than the other. Practice makes it easy and effective.

> Even when you don't wear mascara,
> curl your lashes for the bigger,
> open-eyed look.

Extra lashes are very attractive and a good alternative when lashes are short or thin. Women who use them regularly find they are as easy to put on as lipstick. Placed at the outside corners they give an alluring lift. Be sure to trim to a natural-looking length.

## Lining the Eyes

Lining eliminates the nondescript look, especially if you wear glasses. For a clear, refined line, use an eye lining pen with a fine point or a long-lasting pencil definer. If eyes water, look for waterproof or water-resistant in the labeling.

Liners come in many colors. Brown and black are the most popular. A navy blue liner makes the whites of the eyes whiter, but blue in any eye product draws attention to bluish skin coloration. Brighten topaz shades in brown eyes by using a blue, indigo or navy.

*Application.* Open your mouth slightly to relax the face. If you need more steadiness, rest the elbow on a table with the small finger against your cheek. Trace the color along the roots from the outside corners to the inside.

1.  Upper lids – Look down and gently draw the pen/pencil along the roots of the lashes, but not too close to the inner corners, where color collects. For evening, make the line wider over the pupil of the eye as you look straight into the mirror. Taper the line as it reaches the outer corner. This makes the eyes appear larger.

2.  Lower lids – Look up and draw color along the roots from outer to inner corners, leaving a small space at the inner corners.

3.  If you prefer, line only the outer two-thirds of the upper and/or lower lid.

Lining around the outer eye corners gives a theatrical look and makes eyes look smaller. If you like this effect, be sure it is not too dramatic or too harsh for your face.

## Adding Dimension to Special Eye Shapes

*Close-set Eyes.* (Eyes are close to the bridge of the nose). Place the lightest shade of eye shadow on the inside area and darker shades on the outer area sweeping color up toward outer brow points. Start brow color farther from the nose than the point above the inner eye corner. The arch of your brow should be just beyond the outer edge of the iris. End the brow slightly beyond the outer corner of the eye. Line along the outer two-thirds and extend beyond the outer corner. Use lash-thickening mascara. (See Illustration 8).

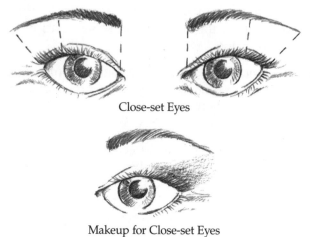

Close-set Eyes

Makeup for Close-set Eyes

Illustration 8

*Wide-set Eyes.* (Eyes are farther from the nose.) Place a shadow, foundation or concealer slightly darker than the skin tone on the inside areas of the eyes and down the side of the nose. Place a deeper shade in the crease of the eye and a lighter one on the outer part. Start brow color closer to the nose than the inside corner and end it above the outer corner. The arch starts in front of the iris. Begin eye lining close to the inner corner and stop before reaching the outer corner. (See Illustration 9.)

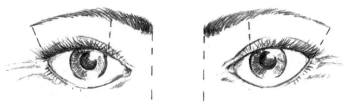

Wide-set Eyes

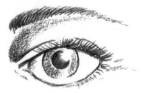

Makeup for Wide-set Eyes

Illustration 9

*Protruding Eyes.* Blend a smoky-to-dark matte shadow from the upper lash line to the crease and slightly beyond the outer corners of the eyes, unless they are wide-set. Use a medium shade from crease to brow with the lightest tone under the brow. A darker brow color "recedes" the protruding lids. Line both the upper and lower lids; smudge for softness. (See Illustration 10.)

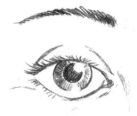
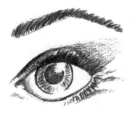

Illustration 10
Makeup for Protruding Eyes

*Deep-set Eyes.* Keep the eyebrow high and arched to give the illusion of more space. Place a light color, ivory or beige, on the lid from the lash line to the crease. Use a muted color, such as taupe or a soft brown, or one that matches your clothing, above the crease and fan to outer brow. This is a triangle of color – from the center of the lid to the outer brow point to the outer corner of the eye. Line outer one-half of lower lids and apply mascara. (See Illustration 11.)

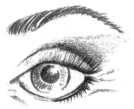

Illustration 11
Makeup for Deep-set Eyes

*Small Eyes.* Blend an ivory or soft taupe eye shadow on upper lids. Use a darker shade from the crease up. Darker color on upper areas between crease and brow makes eyes appear larger, giving an upward focus.

Or, wrap color around
the outside corners.

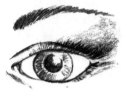

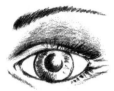

Illustration 12a

Or, form a dome over the center
of each lid by applying a medium-
to-dark shade from lash line to
slightly above crease. Use a pale
shade directly under the brows.

Illustration 12b

Do not use dark shades to line. They "shut in" the eyes. Line the entire upper lid, and rim the lower one from the center to slightly beyond the outer corner.

*Drooping Upper Lids.* Use a pale eye shadow on lids from the lash line to the crease. Place a darker shadow from the lash line to outer brow points, covering the droop. Apply mascara to the outer one-half of the upper and lower lashes and thicker mascara on the lashes in the center of the upper lids. Begin lining from the inner corners and taper off before reaching the outer corner. (See Illustration 13.)

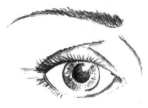

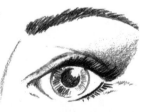

Illustration 13
Camouflaging Drooping
Upper Lids

*Oriental or Asian.* These eyes have minimal lids that may appear to protrude or disappear. For shadow, try the earth tones – taupe, woody browns, olive, grey or charcoal. Blend a medium-toned shadow or foundation to increase the contour from the inner eye up to the inner brow corners. Use a darker shade from the lashes to midway between the lid and brow, then fade the color up toward the brow with the lightest shade directly under the brow. Brush mascara to the outer two-thirds of the lashes. Use an eye lining pen for a delicate trim; trace color along the base of the lashes. (See Illustration 14.)

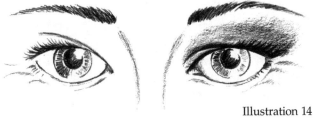

Illustration 14
Makeup for Oriental
or Asian Eyes

## Cosmetic Tattooing

An innovation to adding facial color is permanent cosmetic tattooing of eyebrows, lining eyelids and lips. Softening scars and port wine stains with tattooing has been around a long time. Now, cosmetic tattooing is used to paint permanent brows and line the eyes for women who have lost hair because of aging or breast cancer. It is also used for drawing lifelike nipples on women who have had mastectomies and breast reconstruction.

The growing popularity of cosmetic tattooing is proportional to the increasing number of women past 50 who choose to remain active in work and play. For women whose brows and lashes are sparse or light, and for busy women who are crunching time, tattooing eliminates at least two steps in make-up application. Just think – you can wake up in the morning, get out of the pool, ski or hike, with forever-young brows and defined eyes.

Shapely brows and eye lining via cosmetic tattooing can easily erase years from the face. When done by an artistic expert, they look as natural as the originals, and sometimes better. One woman, who was 84 with failing eyesight, had brows added and lids lined before she became blind.

Cosmetic tattooing can perfect the shape of lips and give them a definite outline and can even eliminate the need to wear lipstick. Cheeks can be tattooed to add color, but generally the result is less than perfect and looks unnatural.

A skilled cosmetic tattooist should have a good educational background in the field and related experience, plus a keen sense of which colors are becoming to a client. It is smart to start with less color because more can always be added. A patch test resolves questions about the right shade. When cosmetic tattooing is done by a qualified technician in the United States, there is little possibility of infection. The skin is anesthetized topically and new sterilized needles are used every time pigment is implanted into the skin.

Because only a few states register cosmetic tattooists, you may need to call your State Board of Cosmetology or a board certified plastic surgeon. Not all states regulate cosmetic tattooing. "Do not go to a body tattooist listed in the classified section of the telephone book," advises Madelyn Stengel, who is registered by the Colorado Board of Cosmetology and is a teacher of cosmetic interdermal tattooing. She is recommended by hospitals, dermatologists and plastic surgeons. Her work involves adding color enhancement to the face, tattooing nipples on reconstructed breasts, and diminishing the appearance of scars on the face and body.

She advises that when you find a cosmetic tattooist, ask for the names of three or four of their clients. Talk to them, observe the work, and look at before and after photographs. After you have talked to the tattooist, ask yourself, Do I like her? Does she understand what I want? Was she easy to talk to and did she take the time to deal with my concerns? Madelyn's advice is be wary, proceed with caution, get what you want not what the tattooist wants, and have realistic expectations.

## Cheeks

Cheer up your cheeks with color! If your choice is to wear very little makeup, blush is imperative. Faces seem lifeless without it. Blush or rouge enlivens the face with color that is naturally associated with health and well-being. It gives sparkle to the eyes by showing off their jewel tones – color reacting with color.

Avoid stripes or dabs of color. Blend blush so that it looks realistic, as though it comes from within. This happens when the complexion is properly primed, tinted with foundation, and the blush shimmers.

Creme blush is usually preferable for dry skin and powder blush for oily, but you can use either one or both. Apply creme rouge, then dust with powder blush for longer-lasting color. Darker shades give more shape to the face than the lighter ones. Creme powder blush stays on the longest.

***Placement.*** Identify the triangle from the top of your ears to the lower edge of the nose to the bottom tip of the ears. Bring the color to the middle of the ear. This is the general area for placement. Now, look straight into the mirror and find the point on the cheekbone directly below the pupil. (See Illustration 15 on page 68.) Blush does not go beyond this point.

Another way to find the proper placement is to use the cheekbone as a guide. Place three dots of color on the cheekbone – at the temple, below the outer edge of your brow and below the center of your eye. Blend toward the middle of the ears. If placed too close to the eye area above the cheekbone, it detracts from the iris and draws attention to puffiness and crow's feet.

*The Long Face.* Keep the blush on the cheekbone to break the vertical line. Blend blush across the lower chin area, a blend not a dab.

*The Wide Face.* Take the color closer to the nose and down to the jawbone at the sides of the face.

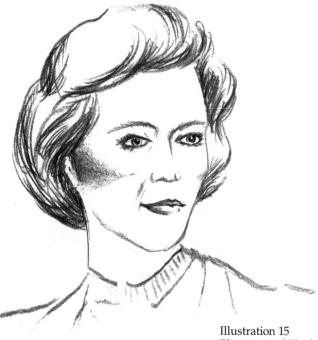

Illustration 15
Placement of Blush

*Fleshy Cheeks.* To get more contour, place a darker shade of blush under the cheekbone, starting down below the outside corners of the eyes and drawing it toward the ears. Blend the edges so the effect, not the technique, is apparent.

*Pointed Chin.* Soften by blending blush under the chin.

*Cheekbones.* Blush placed high on the cheekbones, not in the eye area, emphasizes the contour.

**Eyeglasses.** Blush should glow around the outside corners of the frames.

### Create a Healthy Glow With Blush

- From the point on the cheekbone below the pupil, brush color to the temples, a parenthesis of color around the eyes.

- For the sun-kissed look, sweep it across cheeks and down the nose.

- If you have a high exposed forehead, tint the center just below the hairline.

## Lips

Lip color perks up the whole face with a variety of hues from clear salmon pinks to deep plums, from lush wines to intense berries. Miracles happen with makeup, especially when it comes to lips.

**Lip Lining.** Perfectly-shaped lips are rare, but they appear when properly outlined. Notice the pictures in fashion magazines and see how they have made their lips fuller and shapelier. You can do it, too. A student in a makeup class said she'd had a stroke. One side of her upper lip was lower than the other side. I showed her how to line the lower side higher to match the other side. The correction was easy, and perfected the shape of her lips. (See Illustration 16.)

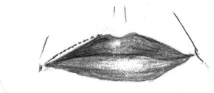

Illustration 16 Lip Lining
to Perfect Shape

A pencil lip liner and sharpener are indispensable. If the point continues to break, return the product and get an automatic lip liner. Always blend lip color into the outlining with a lip brush. When this is not done, the result is unnatural. Dark lip lining with lighter lipstick is too obvious and makes the mouth look hard.

### Tips for Enhancing Your Lips and Face

- For small lips trace, a thin line outside the natural lip border.
- When the borders are uneven, draw them even.
- If one lip is small and the other big, line the small portion outside the border and the larger, inside.
- A round face has better proportion with sharply defined lips.
- A narrow face is softened with fuller, rounder lips.
- If the outer corners droop, uptilt the corners with a wider line above the upper lip corners.

*Lipstick Color.* Light, bright shades make small lips look larger. Dark or muted colors make large lips look smaller. Rich reds or sunny pink-corals de-emphasize a double chin. Some faces look dull without a bright lip color because the undertones of the skin demand vivid shades. If clothing has vibrant tones, makeup should reflect them. Dark clothing colors and evening wear call for a deeper or brighter lip color.

Mixing colors increases your palette. Maybe that color you're not crazy about will be super when combined with another one.

You "soften" the lines surrounding the lips by using a color with a matte, non-shiny finish.

When the bow shape of the upper lip is pronounced, it gives unnecessary sharpness to the mouth. Soften by drawing a line across the lower part of the dip. Fill in with lipstick.

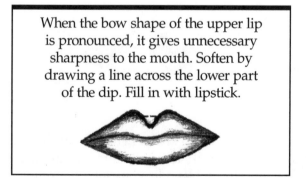

### Application Tips for Longer-Lasting Color

1. Apply a creme foundation around the lip border, stretching the lips across the teeth to get the product into the fine lines. This disguises the lines and covers broken capillaries. Foundation placed on the inside of the lips will cake.

2. Outline as described and press translucent powder on this area.

3. Fill in with a lip brush rather than the lipstick itself. This gives a thinner coat which lasts longer than a thick coat. Use a light color on a thin upper lip (to make it appear fuller) and a darker shade on a full lower lip (to make it thinner) or vice versa for symmetry. Blot.

4. Lipstick brands with a stain or fewer emollients stay on better.

*Feathering.* When lip color seeps into the fine lines around the mouth and looks smeared, it is called feathering or bleeding. The gradual loss of collagen in this area causes a blurring of the border between the lip and the skin, but don't despair. Here are some ways to restrain wandering color.

- Moisturizers with collagen temporarily plump up the lines.
- Apply a lip conditioner or primer before your color.
- Be sure to get your foundation in the lines around the lips. Creme or powder creme foundation fills in the lines better than liquid foundation.
- Outlining the lips holds the color in.
- Some lipsticks are advertised as non-bleeding.
- A dermatologist can inject collagen into the lines and redefine the lip border because the procedure adds lost volume to thinning lips. Touch-ups are required every six months or so.

*Flaky Lips.* Dab petroleum jelly onto moist lips. Gently slough away flakes with a soft tooth brush or dry terry washcloth. An alpha hydroxy acid product may also help this condition.

## African American, Hispanic and Asian Skin___

If you have never played up your color with flattering makeup, do it now! Realize your beauty potential.

*Skin Care.* Use nonirritating products, alcohol/fragrance free and oil-free if skin is oily. Exfoliation or masking is important. Moisturize dry areas, especially around the eyes where wrinkles show up first. All skin types need sun protection. Use a nonsensitizing product.

*Foundation.* Use one that is water-based, oil-free and covers well. The shade should match skin tones exactly and brighten the eyes. If necessary, mix two in your palm to get the best color.

*Translucent Powder.* Powder adds warmth, prevents an ashy look and minimizes shine by absorbing excess oil. The shade should be very close to the tone of your foundation. Powdering gives a matte finish. Blot with blotting papers when oil appears and dust again.

*Cheeks and Lips.* Warm or cool skin tones determine your best color choices. Some suggestions are: For lighter skin coral, mauve, red, amber. For medium-tones – rose, brick, copper, russet. For ebony – wine, bronze, burgundy, dark red. To tone down red, mix with tinted lip gloss or foundation.

To make full lips smaller, line the lips inside the normal lip border with a raisin or burgundy lip liner. Fill in with a dark shade of lipstick.

*Eyes.* They are the windows of your soul and the mirror of your personality. Eyes with added color are more expressive. If you wear glasses, use heavier liner, shadow and mascara.

*Shadow.* For black brown irises use black, dark brown, navy blue, dark green, purple, rust, or mauve. For other eye colors see the previous section on Eye Shadow, Guidelines for Selecting Eye Shadow Colors, page 58. When a color is too bright, tone it down with brown or beige.

*Shadow Highlighters.* Depending upon your skin tone, use golden-bronze, beige, pale mauve, violet, dusty pink. When you have few or no lines, add glamour to evening wear with the metallic glint of gold, bronze or copper in the outer corner of the brows or the outside corner of your cheekbone. Carefully blend.

*Lining the Eyes.* When black is harsh, use grey or brown. For more color use dark blue, wine or purple, especially if they imitate clothing colors. When the whites take on a yellowish hue, avoid brown. It intensifies the yellow. Gray, black and midnight blue will brighten the yellowish look.

## *Makeovers*

All women are over 50. The photos are not retouched to conceal lines or wrinkles. As in my Magic of Makeup classes, the women applied their own makeup with my guidance. For all three, I added brow color above the inner points to restore the youthful lift. In the "after" pictures, they wear a quality foundation that gives good coverage.

> With care, color and know-how, we can take age out of image.

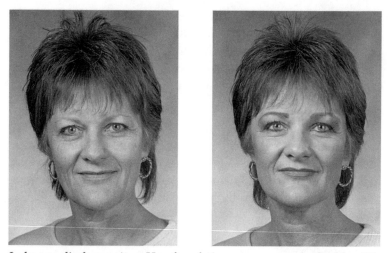

Judy—medical recruiter. Her foundation even conceals freckles. We enriched her eyes with brow color and black lash-thickening mascara. She always lines her eyes ... calls it her "trademark." Lining the eyes makes the whites whiter. Eye shadow is shades of brown. We drew lips fuller with a lip definer pencil and filled in with a rich red.

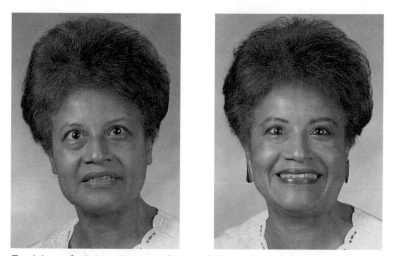

Patricia—administration coordinator. We used an ivory concealant to lighten eye areas, extended and darkened the brows with black brow pencil, then used black mascara and shadow with black eye liner. Blush was blended from the upper ear tip to mid-ear and lower ear tip to directly below the pupils on the cheek bone. Her smile adds sparkle to her eyes.

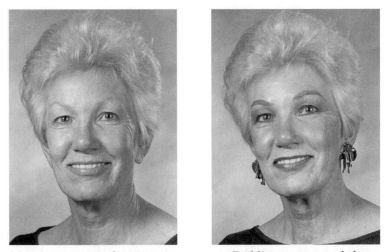

Margaret—owner of an insurance agency. Ruddiness was toned down with a concealant before applying foundation. We added width and color to brows with a taupe brow pencil and eye shadow in tones of brown diminishing darker shade to above the brow bone. She has full lips with deep color and gets the best shade by using an underbase before she applies a medium shade of lip color. Unlike Judy and Patricia, blush is shaped parallel with check bones to balance facial length—not triangular as described for Patricia.

## *The Professional Finish*

Translucent powder is fine-textured and available in different shades. It can be pressed, as in compacts, or loose. Pressed powder is tops for touchups and zapping T-zone shine. Keep loose powder for home use. This sheer powder offsets the shine of some moisturizing foundations that may exaggerate lines. Shine shows up lines! It helps makeup to last longer and softens/blends colors. If it dulls them, especially blush, you have applied too much.

Go light on powdering. Dust the facial hairs down with a brush and minimal powder. If powder collects in lines, it emphasizes them. Some powders draw oil and moisture from the skin. On dry skin, even a light dusting with translucent powder may settle in the lines or accentuate a flaky texture.

Women with dry skin may prefer to mist their face by using a commercial spray, such as Evian. They have one that fits in your purse. Besides adding a dewy get-up and glow, it "sets" the makeup for dry skin the way powder does for combination and oily skin.

For the working woman, a midday dewy spritz hydrates thirsty skin and will not muss makeup. The small atomizer is also handy for women who travel and experience dehydration.

## Makeup for the Occasion

The occasion and the time of day influence how, and what makeup we should wear. Keep the face attractive and timeless whether the occasion is casual or formal. When participating in exercise classes, athletics, hiking, etc., wear minimal makeup. I was on a group hike and one of the women wore eye makeup suitable for a cocktail party. By the end of the hike her shadow was spotty and her eye lining was smearing. She looked worn-out. Maybe she was, but the runaway makeup didn't help.

Minimal makeup still looks finished. For sheer base color, try one of the following:

- Your regular liquid foundation
- Equal parts of foundation and a moisturizer
- A liquid foundation formulated with a moisturizer
- A moisturizer with a tint
- A self-tanning oil or lotion

Then add brow color, blush and a trace of lipstick. If you have good lip pigmentation, you may want only a touch of lip gloss. For small pale lips, rim with lip liner and add color.

If you are going from work or an afternoon activity to an evening engagement, deepen your daytime colors. To dramatize the eyes with shadow, sweep it subtly from the outer corners up toward the temples to give more lift. Maybe you want a wedge of shadow or eye lining around the outer eye corners. Give blush a dash more color and redo the lips. Nighttime colorings are more daring and satiny than daytime.

> Avoid being a fade-out. Promise yourself to touch-up makeup midday, mid-evening, mid-occasion, whenever necessary and convenient. Most makeup fades in two to three hours, depending on the oiliness of the skin and the quality of the product.

## *Do's and Don'ts*

Do get an enriching foundation, enriching in color. When you apply a foundation that is the same color as your complexion, many times the result is a wash-out. Try one shade darker and notice the difference. If this slightly darker shade has the same undertones as your skin, it will not contrast with the skin on your throat.

Do extend brow color to the outer point of the brows. Do not stop midway.

Don't let brows pop up like EKG ratings. Add color to heighten the inner points.

Don't put up with skimpy brows. Fatten them up!

Don't use thick eye lining that reminds us of raccoons. It detracts from the beauty of the eyes and the whole face. Use a narrow defining line.

Don't put on so much mascara that it sheds below the eyes.

Don't wear garish eye shadow or loud lipstick or any color that shouts for attention unless you really are a clown!

Do make blush a blend, not a dab. Use a larger brush.

Do wear lip color. Lining your lips perfects their shape and lip color vitalizes the face.

Do touch up lipstick after eating. You don't have to look like a faded rose.

Do a disappearing act on the double chin as shown in Illustration 17. Dust a bronzer or tawny-colored blush just beneath the jawbone and chin. A classic red lip color minimizes a double chin.

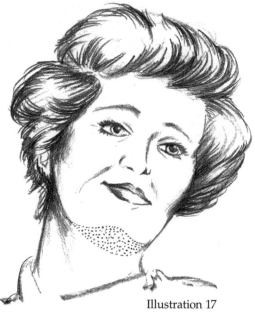

Illustration 17
Contouring for the Double Chin

Do blot excess oil without disturbing makeup. Try Goody end papers for perms available at drugstores, 500 for a couple dollars.

Do check your face in daylight before you leave home and make corrections.

Do remember: Wearing makeup is not vain. It gives the same pleasure as seeing petunias and geraniums in full bloom. More than that, the good feeling that goes with the realization that beauty beyond 50 is possible puts poise in our demeanor, a sparkle in our eyes and a spring in our step.

## Excess Facial Hair

After 40, women grow more facial hair and sometimes a few coarse ones because of changes in the hormonal balance. During a makeup class, one woman exclaimed, "Just look at all the hair on my face! I'm so embarrassed by it. It's terrible!" She was surprised to find that no one else had noticed this "terrible" hair. People view us from at least three feet away and seldom see the things that make us self-conscious.

Tweeze the few coarse hairs. Warm wax removal of superfluous hair is easy and quick. The only discomfort is a momentary smarting when the wax is pulled off. With this process the hair grows back fine and soft without a stubble. Regrowth takes four to six weeks. This is a job for the professional, not the amateur. Hot wax removal can cause a second degree burn. The wax has to be the right temperature and the skin must be held a certain way when removing the wax. Many salons and beauty schools offer this service. The cost at beauty schools is reasonable. Some have senior discounts.

After several professional treatments, you may feel you know the procedure well enough to try a cold wax removal and do it yourself. A chemical or wax depilatory removes the hair at the surface. Within a few days stubble can be seen and felt. To avoid this, find a product that removes the hair at the roots and follow the manufacturer's instructions.

Guaranty Hair Removal No-Needle Electrolysis™ has FDA approved labeling for permanent hair removal. This process causes no scar tissue, scabs or nerve damage because there is no penetration into the skin. For women of color this means there is *no* change in skin tone. "When the epidermis layer of the skin is punctured, there is a possibility of infection, disease or scarring. The GHR process kills the hair follicle without invading the body and leaves no scar or change in pigmentation regardless of skin color. We can remove hair permanently from any part of the body," said Judith G. Stephens, MS, Certified Clinical Electrologist and inventor of the GHR device.

The procedure involves softening the hair with a cleansing and treatment solution that creates receptivity to electrical current. The operator then grips it with a tweezer and applies direct current that travels down the shaft to the root, permanently decomposing it. Some body hair requires more than one treatment. Tweezing nose hairs can lead to staph infection, so it is better to clip them or use the GHR No-Needle Electrolysis™.

GHR is affordable for the average person and is tax deductible *if* it is used for improving psychological and physiological well-being, such as hair on chin, upper lip, chest or ingrown hairs. Call 1-800-833-4471 to get more details. They will tell you where the GHR treatment is obtainable in your area.

## Stay Up-to-Date!

How many times have we wished we had someone's opinion on new ideas we want to try? If you have one or two good friends and you like the way they do their faces, get together and experiment with different techniques or colors. Maybe they want advice, too. Take advantage of every opportunity to learn about makeup.

Pictures in women's magazines illustrate the current modes of facial design. Even if the models are young, you can mimic the makeup applications that fit your style. Browsing through women's magazines, you find out what is current and what may be worth buying in the world of cosmetics. Occasionally, there are articles about makeovers, surveys of new products, and advice from experts on hair, makeup, and skin care as well as helpful information from models and celebrities.

Working with different colorings and placements stimulates your creativity. You will catch yourself thinking, "I wonder how this would look?" Be caring about your face. Individualize the makeup tips in this chapter and you will look as young as you feel. Stay with a simple and uncomplicated routine. You will see how makeup magnifies your winning image.

> The intelligent and caring woman who is over 50 wears makeup. It is smart because the aging face with artful makeup comes alive. It is caring when we present our best face to friends, relatives, and the people we meet.

# 4

# You Can Brighten Your Smile

> "So your hair's falling out, and your
> cute little father has just switched from
> Chaplin revivals to porno flicks,
> And your orthodontist recommends
> braces—immediately...
> You might as well laugh."
> —Judith Viorst, *Forever Fifty*[1]

You will laugh heartier and oftener with white, even-looking teeth. We don't have to tolerate telltale yellow or crooked teeth and it's healthier not to. Straightening enables us to maintain the long-term health of teeth and gums and to keep the jaw line age-resistant. Both whitening and straightening give us the physical and psychological lift of an attractive, pleasing smile. It's not as hard as you may think.

"Our faces and facial expressions are two of the truest reflections of the way we feel about ourselves." Tom Linnell, a psychologist practicing in Ft. Collins, Colorado said. "If we have to hide our faces in embarrassment, it means we're also hiding part of ourselves. Being able to smile openly brightens our whole personality."[2]

## Whitening

Dull, dingy teeth can be transformed into a shiny, youthful white according to Donald L. Finks, D.D.S. of Denver, Colorado. Unsmiling women with yellowing teeth find new freedom of expression when they are whitened. It literally changes personalities. "A smile says much more than words," Dr. Finks said. "It expresses the warmth of an individual's personality and makes a remarkable difference." For women who associate with people on a career or service basis, a sparkling smile is a big asset. It's an asset for any active woman.

Stains are classified as two kinds. Extrinsic stains result from cigarettes, cigars, coffee, tea, red wine, and some medications. These are easier to remove than intrinsic stains that are incorporated into the enamel and will not lighten as well.

The process does not replace daily oral hygiene and regular professional cleaning. Simple and painless, it consists of wearing clear plastic guards or trays that are customized to fit the teeth and contain a bleaching gel. The bleaching component is a 10 percent solution of carbamide peroxide which has been used for years as an oral antiseptic. The trays can be worn on either the uppers or lowers or both from bedtime to awakening. Eighty to 100 hours of soaking teeth in the bleaching gel is required, depending on the nature of the discoloration. After five or six nights, teeth can be four shades lighter. There is no way to predict exact results. One year after the initial whitening, a touchup for several nights is advised. If you smoke or drink, restaining occurs quicker and you will need touchups more often.

Whitening is easier on the pocketbook than capping, bonding or veneers. Compared to these, it is a relatively inexpensive way to have an attractive smile at any age. Cost may range from $200 to $400. This is just one of the many facets of the large and rapidly growing field of cosmetic dentistry. The dental society in your area has a referral service to help you find doctors in this field.

Teeth aren't extracted now as often as they were in past decades. It's no longer a fact that dentures are in our future. Dr. Finks has patients in their 70s and 80s – one is 96 – who still have their own teeth. This is the trend. Denture wearers take three times longer to masticate their food than people who have their originals. With regular dental hygiene and daily brushing, the majority of people are expected to keep their teeth for a lifetime, and they can be pearly white, too.

## Straightening

Many people past 40 are having their teeth straightened because of longstanding discomfort, teeth moving into peculiar positions, or they are just fed up with the embarrassment of crooked teeth. To hide imperfect alignment people adopt mannerisms or never smile. Today, men and women over 40, 50, even 60 and 70, are asking: Why not straighten those teeth that have bothered me all these years? Orthodontia for this group has tripled since the 1980s. Almost everyone I talked with knew someone over 40 who had their teeth straightened, or they themselves had done it. Amazingly few of us are born with perfect teeth.

As my bite worsened, and after the second grandchild, I began to consider doing something about it. The thought of a steely smile kept putting me off, so I asked friends, What do you think about my wearing braces? Without exception, the replies were, Do it! They all knew at least one person over 40 who was happy with orthodontic correction.

In my quest for more confirmation, I talked with women who had tested the waters. Betty, a supervisor and landsman with an oil company, said the year she turned 50 was depressing the whole twelve months. Facing increased competition from younger personnel and wanting a business career for 15 to 20 more years, she realized self-improvement was imperative. She lost 15 pounds and whittled her figure into shape. Then, she had her upper teeth capped and at 55, the lower ones were straightened. Since her teen years, she had always been self-conscious about her mouth. One tooth actually sat sideways. This was corrected by wearing braces for six months and a retainer for a year.

She was amazed at how easy and efficient the correction was and wished she had done it years before "because it turned out to be such a simple thing." There is no question in her mind that a youthful, healthy appearance is important on the professional scene.

Ellie, a woman in her 70s, said her lower teeth were moving in such a way that they lacerated her lip. When she decided to have them straightened, her husband thought she was crazy and asked, "What's an old woman like you straightening her teeth for?" In eight months her teeth were even, and she had experienced no pain or discomfort with the braces. Only the habitual brushing three times a day was bothersome. If she hadn't done it, her lower teeth would still be cutting her lip. Not only did her teeth look a lot better, but her gums were healthier.

When I came back from the orthodontist's office with the metallic contraptions on, I was surprised when someone said, "You look younger!" and another thought I looked "cute!" Besides the association of braces with the very young, the brackets plumped out the lines around my lips. My mouth felt cluttered, and I didn't want to smile that first week, let alone eat. My daughter advised me not to worry because it only attracted more attention, and "Besides," she said, "they're not that noticeable."

Most of the people who commented about them had either worn braces, knew people over 40 who had, or wished their teeth were straighter. It was exciting to see the teeth moving into line and realize that for the first time in my life I was going to have a smile that didn't have a tinge of self-consciousness.

Dr. Daryl R. Burns, D.D.S., has been practicing orthodontics for 37 years and his current patients include children and young people and several who are 40 to 80 years old. He said repositioning teeth in adulthood takes longer and is not as easy or efficient as it is in childhood. Successful corrections can certainly be completed after midlife.

Coequal to the advantage of straight teeth is the re-education in oral hygiene, an indispensable part of the orthodontic procedure. The American Dental Association contends that, with good oral hygiene, your teeth can last a lifetime.[3]

Besides the cosmetic advantage, straight teeth contribute to dental health. They are easier to clean, and there's less stress to the surrounding tissues. This means a reduction in the risk of teeth loosening, gum disease, and the loss of gum, bone, or teeth.

For the duration of the treatment, the patient must punctuate the day with brushings, flossing and the use of a flushing machine. A flushing machine shoots a pulsating current of water that washes out particles between the teeth that are not probed by brushing. The force of the spray massages the gums and leaves a squeaky-clean mouth. Conscientious orthodontic clients probably have the cleanest mouths in town, and the pleasantness is likely to make the routine permanent.

To meet the requirements for orthodontic treatment, the patient must be highly motivated – willing to put time into the cleansing routine in order to have healthy teeth, gums, and bone. If the teeth and braces are not kept clean, gum tissues could become inflamed. There is the risk of root resorption or of a tooth becoming non-vital from movement. These problems don't occur very often because periodic x-rays and frequent examinations of gum tissue prevent them. Present-day appliances with resilient wires, not rigid and tough as they used to be, also reduce risk. Pain is inconsequential in modern orthodontia.

The biggest bugaboo is vanity. Fortunately, the industry has come out with porcelain brackets that are clear with flesh-colored ties. Some of the self-consciousness of a metallic grin is removed with these new appliances. This is a small inconvenience compared to the enduring advantages of a healthy bite and even teeth.

According to Dr. Burns, straight teeth and oral hygiene aren't the total answer to dental health. They must be combined with checkups and a diet that gives the teeth plenty of exercise through chewing fresh fruits and vegetables.

Dr. Burns said that straight teeth "build up one's self-confidence to have a smile that goes from ear to ear. There are lots of people walking around who do not smile because their teeth are irregular. When you converse with someone, it's a great feeling to know you have an even set of teeth."

---

For healthy teeth and a bright smile,
brush for one minute –
count one to 60 – and floss daily.

# 5

# Erasing the Wrinkles and Breast Reduction

"I've never liked the way I looked
and you know what that does to
your self-esteem. [At 71] I've never
looked so good in my entire life."
—Phyllis Diller[1] (after many
facial and dental corrections)

The unceasing flow of good easy-to-do ideas on how to maintain good mental and physical health increases the likelihood of a 100-year lifespan. The years after 50 can be filled with different occupations, careers, service, fun and adventure. Nowadays most women have two vocations – one as homemaker and the other outside the home. It's not unusual for women to spend several years in one line of work and then reeducate themselves for something entirely different. Longevity is acceptable and welcome if it is enriched with useful activity, good health and a pleasing appearance.

## Erasing the Wrinkles

It's no news that a double standard persists in today's society: Wrinkles are okay for men but not for women. That's one reason why women want to mute as many wrinkles as they can. A better reason is that women enjoy life more if they like what they see in the mirror. If eliminating a few lines and wrinkles or other unsightly aberrations – surgically or topically – relieves chronic unhappiness (a very real malady), the money is well spent. Overhauling the skin can be very gratifying. It's far healthier than withdrawing into depression.

An important follow-up is to nourish the skin with routine maintenance or unattractive textures will gradually reappear. Beneficial eating and planned physical activity should also be a day-by-day lifestyle.

## Retin-A

Retin-A is a synthetic derivative of vitamin A acid (tretinoin). This prescriptive drug, patented and manufactured by Ortho Pharmaceutical Corporation, a division of Johnson & Johnson, is available in a gel, creme or liquid. Renova is an excellent creme and costs about $20 a month.

Many users receive compliments on the lovely results. Years seem to drop away from their face. Retin-A diminishes lines and wrinkles, smooths rough areas, and lightens age spots. It gives the skin more even pigmentation and a dewy glow. The process normalizes the skin by thinning the thick top epidermal layer and restoring the lower epidermal layer to normal thickness. It does not help with deep furrows or sagging skin.

According to Dr. Barbara Reed, a dermatologist and enthusiastic user, success of topical treatments depends to a large extent upon the type of skin. For example, oily skin is easier to treat than thin, very dry, or ruddy skin. Women who are sun lovers or who have eczema or very sensitive skin should not use it. Acne-prone women may experience a temporary flair-up that gradually disappears.

At first there may be a burning sensation. Applying too much may result in scaliness and redness. This is remedied by not using it for a few days. Be careful when applying it to the corners of the mouth, nose, around the eyes and other sensitive areas. Because the treatment makes the skin very dry and super sensitive to the sun, wind and cold, an SPF 15 or greater sunscreen and moisturizer are indispensable.

Continual use of tretinoin is necessary to retain the benefits. A good routine is to apply it in the evening. In the morning, put on a sunscreen, then moisturize. Although improvement is visible within a few weeks, it takes six to 12 months or longer to see the full effect. After this time, fewer applications are required.

## Laser Resurfacing

The forces of longevity and science have united to make possible the smoothing away of aging and sun-damaged skin, leaving healthier, younger looking skin. Skin resurfacing with laser light gives a smooth complexion without the pain, inconvenience or expense of surgery, electrocautery, freezing, sanding or other traditional treatments. Some patients have said it is not as bad as going to the dentist. Eventually, laser techniques may replace many current cosmetic surgical procedures.

"I am very enthusiastic about this procedure because it has a risk factor of less than one percent without cutting, bleeding, or chemicals. Consequently, the risk of scarring or pigmentation problems is greatly reduced. Laser resurfacing has repeatedly provided safe predictable results," said Richard G. Asarch, M.D. Asarch is board certified in both dermatology and dermatopathology, a Fellow in the American Society for Laser Medicine and Surgery, and Associate Clinical Professor of Dermatology at the University of Colorado Health Sciences Center.

Tremendous advances in laser technology permit lasers to be used for resurfacing. Successful results have been produced on men and women of all skin types, ages and ethnicities, but the lighter the skin, the more pleasing the results. There is less damage to surrounding tissues, little patient discomfort and swelling, better depth control, more consistent results and a relatively short recovery time.

Such a high recommendation cannot always be given to dermabrasion or chemical peels where the risk factor is greater and changes in pigmentation may occur. Dermabrasion involves bleeding and often a slower, more uncomfortable post-operative period. With chemical peels it is difficult to control the depth of chemical penetration and changes in skin color. However, the laser is not used for sagging or loose skin, deep lines, the throat area, or dark circles under the eyes. These are corrected with other procedures.

Laser surgery permanently removes spots, birthmarks, acne and chickenpox scars, precancerous lesions, rosacea (redness), stretch marks, unwanted blemishes and benign growths. The treatment removes the "crinkled" skin beneath the lower eyelids, the "crow's feet" around the eyes and lines around the mouth. It is the best treatment for treating acne scars. Some lasers stimulate collagen production resulting in younger looking skin. Like any surgery, the patient has to be psychologically prepared.

Laser machines cost in the ballpark of $125,000, hence the treatment is expensive. Cost varies from $500 to $5,000 depending upon the city where your doctor practices and whether you have just one area treated, such as the forehead, eyes, cheeks, lips, or the entire face. Insurance does not cover aesthetic laser surgery. As of this writing, it does cover precancerous lesions.

Different laser machines are used for different conditions. The **Nd:YAG laser**, when used with a topical carbon emulsion, removes facial and body hairs. The **tunable dye laser** erases age spots from the backs of the hands and spider veins. The **pulse dye laser** is primarily used for birthmarks, spider veins on the face, and the underlying redness of acne rosacea. Results from this laser are instantaneous but skin appears darkened for 10 to 14 days. The **photoderm light device** has almost no side effects or darkening. It is especially good for spider veins on the legs.

With the **carbon dioxide laser** old looking or sun damaged skin is dramatically reduced layer-by-layer with a degree of tightening to reduce wrinkles. It works well for vertical lines around the mouth, crow's-feet near the eyes, and lines on the cheeks. Using a device like an artist's brush, a doctor can "paint" away lines around the eyes and the mouth. Tattoos and some brown freckles vanish. It is not as effective on smile lines or deep forehead wrinkles. Research indicates that it increases the production of collagen and elastin. Because it removes the top layer of the dermis, crusting forms.

The laser produces a high energy invisible beam of light that is absorbed by water in the skin cells and causes vaporization of tissue. It feels like a rubber band snapping against the skin. Because laser resurfacing involves no bleeding or chemicals to cover the surface, the treatment area is clearly visible. This allows pinpoint precision. It is performed in the doctor's office during one sitting, under local anesthesia with or without mild sedation. A small area takes a few minutes, the entire face about two hours. Healing takes from seven to 14 days. Redness occurs afterwards and takes longer to disappear, in some cases several months. New medications are speeding up this process but it will be necessary to wear makeup until it disappears. To protect the healthy new skin, the patient must wear a sunscreen with an SPF of at least 15 at all times.

On rare occasions, problems may occur following treatment, such as some scarring, infection and changes in skin color. They are not common but they have occurred. Lasers do not produce X-ray radiation but protective glasses are required in the laser treatment room.

Do the following to ensure good results:

■ Make sure the doctor is skillful and experienced in skin-resurfacing laser surgery who owns the machine and does not rent it. Call the American Society for Dermatologic Surgery, (708) 330-9830, to find an experienced doctor in your area.

■ When you go in for a consultation, ask to see "before and after" photos and talk to patients the doctor has treated.

This will give you additional information and down-to-earth tips. Ask questions. No question is stupid when you need assurance. For example:

What is the total cost for what I want done?
What should I expect during and after the process?
Is it damaging to the eyes, nose or other sensitive areas?
Do I wear bandages afterwards? What will my face look like after the treatment and after it has healed?

- Advise your physician of any history of cold sores or herpes outbreak. They will prescribe preventive medications.

- Plan to take one to two weeks off from work for recuperation.

- Follow the instructions you receive for care and treatment during and after the healing process. Do not use cosmetics/makeup the first week after the procedure. Your physician will give you a specific antibiotic ointment and compresses to use during this critical time. What little crusting does occur can be lessened by keeping the surface moist during the healing process. Skin can be sensitive for several three months. During this time avoid sun exposure to prevent brown discoloration, particularly if you have an olive skin tone.

- When the crusting is gone, the following is recommended:

A cleanser for dry sensitive skin
Moisturizing oil
Non-chemical sunscreen with SPF 15
Liquid makeup with sunscreen SPF 15
Extra rich face cream if your skin needs it

(Dr. Lynda Sý, a dermatologist in Lafayette, California, has developed products and a regimen for post-laser care. They are sold in dermatologists' offices or you may call 800-232-3376 if you reside in California, or 800-422-3376 if you live in another state.)

Because nothing prevents wrinkling or aging, laser resurfacing can be repeated in five to 10 years for the professional whose career demands an upbeat appearance and for anyone who wants an ageless face that reflects her active lifestyle. Living to 80 or 90 will become more and more common, so this is a sensible and uplifting option. After laser resurfacing, one woman said, "No matter how old we get we still care about the face we present....It's an elevation [to my well being] when I look the best I can."

## Face-lift (Rhytidectomy)

Some results of the aging of the skin can only be remedied by plastic surgery. (The derivation of the word "plastic" is the Greek word, "plastikos," meaning molding or giving form.) It is the only procedure that corrects deep wrinkles, pouches on the sides of the mouth, jowls and the wrinkling, fleshy throat. Rhytidectomy (surgical face-lifting), dermabrasion (rubbing away skin aberrations), skin peeling (acid applications) and collagen injections are used in plastic surgery.

Whether to have a face-lift is a question that warrants careful, longterm evaluation. Consider the risks and the benefits and talk to women who have had them. Definite improvement is possible, but women who expect perfection are often disappointed. A bad face-lift or one that is too taut, changing the expression, calls attention to itself but good work is virtually undetectable. Jacqueline Kennedy Onassis had multiple lifts yet did not look overprocessed.

If plastic surgery is your choice, find a qualified and capable plastic surgeon by:

- Consulting your family physician or internist
- Calling the local County Medical Society
- Asking the local teaching or first class community hospital
- Writing the Executive Office of the American Society of Plastic and Reconstructive Surgeons, Inc., 444 E. Algonquin Road, Arlington Heights, IL 60005, or phone (800) 635-0635, the Patient Referral Service. Or, the American Board of Medical Specialties (800) 776-2378

- Visiting the library and checking the *Directory of Medical Specialists* published by Marquis' Who's Who, Inc. or the American Board of Medical Specialties' *Compendium of Certified Medical Specialists.*

Be wary of exaggerated and sensational claims in the news media or so-called "cosmetic surgeons" who are not board certified and whose training is not as comprehensive. They use a hard-sell approach and may brush aside your concerns about safety.

Physicians certified by the American Board of Plastic Surgery must pursue postgraduate training of five to seven years. It includes thorough grounding in general surgery and a minimum of two to three years in an approved plastic surgery training center. In addition, they must pass a rigorous examination to be officially certified by the American Board of Plastic Surgery or its Canadian equivalents, the Royal College of Physicians and Surgeons of Canada or the Corporation Professionelle du Medicin de Quebec.

The American Board of Plastic Surgery is the only board approved by the American Board of Medical Specialties for determining qualifications and certification in plastic surgery. The certification of a physician by the American Board of Plastic Surgery does not guarantee perfect results. Medicine is an inexact art and postoperative results are dependent upon several factors, which are sometimes unpredictable. The more thorough the surgeon's training, skill and experience, the greater the possibility that results will be satisfying.

Responsible doctors do not mind answering these questions:

- Where do you have hospital privileges? Generally, this assures that the doctor has been reviewed by his or her peers.

- How safe is this operation?

- What are the potential side effects of the surgical procedure and how long will they last? Patients should know the side effects to decide when they can resume normal activities.

- How much will this cost?

- How many of your patients have needed additional surgery to correct problems occurring from the original operation? The patient needs to know the probability of more surgical correction and if there will be an additional charge.

- May I contact former patients who have had the same surgical procedure that I want?

- What should I expect before, during, and after the operation?

- If the doctor is unwilling to answer all of your concerns, find one who will.[2]

Betty, the woman pictured on the cover of my first book and whose photo precedes the Epilogue in this edition is an elegant 5'7" longtime fashion model. At 55, she was forced to either stop working or do something about her aging face. Her gynecologist recommended a board certified plastic surgeon. During the consultation the surgeon explained exactly what had to be done and the risks. Because her health was good and her enthusiasm and determination high, she was a good candidate.

Risk is always present when you are on the operating table for five hours but they are reduced when you have a competent surgeon. Although healing can take as long as six months, Betty healed fast. Two weeks later she was on a modeling assignment. She only had a little puffiness around the eyes and it soon disappeared. The biggest advantage to her was to be able to continue her career.

For healthy skin she follows a skin care regimen and takes plenty of vitamins A, C, E and kelp. Her advice is to be very selective when choosing a doctor, and to "go for it when you are mentally prepared." Psychological preparation is crucial. Do it for yourself, not for your husband or anyone else. Feeling good about appearance ensures self-confidence and the perks that come from heightened self-esteem. Betty said. "It may not get a husband or a dream job, but there will be more possibilities."

A successful face-lift is the result of a well-prepared patient with the correct motivation, realistic expectations, anatomical characteristics of skin that are conducive to surgery, and an expertly executed procedure. Dr. George M. Lacy, who is board certified, said that during a consultation the patient's motivation, physical condition, and medical history are discussed. He explains the appropriate corrective procedure, expectations and risks. Tanning, smoking, drinking, and weight affect the way faces heal. If a client has unresolved medical complications, or neurotic or psychotic problems, a doctor may refuse to perform surgery.

The psychological element involved in evaluating the patient for cosmetic surgery is important both before and after surgery. "We don't get involved in psychotherapy, but the way a patient looks at herself both before and after surgery is very important," Dr. Lacy said. A woman who is depressed because she looks haggard and wants to reenter the job market or have more social life is a good candidate.

In any type of surgery there are statistical risks, such as bleeding, infection, unusual scar formation, and poor healing. This can happen even when the operation is properly done by a well-trained surgeon in a correct environment on a qualified patient. But, Dr. Lacy emphasized, usually everything usually works out fine, and the patient is pleased with the results.

In Dr. Lacy's opinion, "The three most harmful things that affect the skin over the years are overexposure to the sun, smoking and any overindulgence." Harmful exposure to the sun and smoking are the worst. Persons who tan heavily destroy many elastic fibers in the face. They are more likely to have crinkly parchment-like skin as they age.

"We know that patients who smoke don't do as well with a face-lift, or any kind of surgery, particularly skin flap surgery. A face-lift does involve large skin flaps. In the smoker, the blood supply to the skin and face is significantly decreased, and the incidence of impaired circulation resulting in crusting, death of skin in the skin flaps, and excessive scarring is higher. This has become such a well-known fact. While most plastic surgeons won't necessarily refuse to do a smoker, almost all insist that the patient quit smoking at least one week before and one week after the operation."

Changes created by a successful face-lift are subtle. Usually, a woman has only one and maybe periodic tucks. The amount of relifting differs with each client, depending upon the quality of her skin, the amount of fat under the skin, facial shape and the type of initial surgery.

It is important to protect the new complexion by conscientiously following the doctor's skin care advice, especially for the first six to 10 weeks. This includes a gentle water soluble cleanser, a moisturizer and SPF 15 sunscreen. Plastic surgeons say that women who learn how to apply makeup realize a greater return on their investment than those who don't.

## The "Spiritual Face-lift"

Dr. Maxwell Maltz, one of the world's best-known plastic surgeons, wrote in his bestseller, *Psycho-Cybernetics:*

"Try giving yourself a 'Spiritual Face-lift.' It is more than a play on words. It opens you up to more life, more vitality, the 'stuff' that youth is made of. You'll feel younger. You'll actually look younger. Many times I have seen a man or woman apparently grow five or 10 years younger in appearance after removing old emotional scars. Look around you. Who are the youthful-looking people you know over the age of forty? The grumpy? Resentful? The pessimistic? The ones who are 'soured on the world,' or the cheerful, optimistic, good-natured people?

"Carrying a grudge against someone or against life can bring on the old age stoop, just as much as carrying a heavy weight around on your shoulders would. People with emotional scars, grudges, and the like are living in the past, which is characteristic of old people. The youthful attitude and youthful spirit erases wrinkles from the soul and the face... looks to the future and has a great expectation....

"So why not give yourself a face-lift? Your do-it-yourself kit consists of relaxation of negative tensions to prevent scars... creative living, a willingness to be a little vulnerable, and a nostalgia for the future instead of the past."[*3]

## Breast Reduction (Reduction Mammaplasty) _____

Many women tolerate oversized breasts their whole life and then after 50 they get even larger. Here is a remedy they can look into even if they have to borrow the money to do it. The resulting relief is as great as the pleasure of a new car or a new home, and it is felt every waking moment in a woman's life.

These women experience many medical problems. They can have unflagging neck and back pain, irritation to skeletal deformities, osteoarthritis of the cervical spine, and breathing problems. Bra straps may leave indentations in their shoulders. Unusually large breasts make women feel self-conscious. They become round-shouldered. Consequently, breast reduction is usually performed to get freedom from physical discomfort and restriction of activities rather than for cosmetic reasons. Besides eliminating excessive weight and improving posture, it gives a psychological lift.

Dr. Robert Hoehn, M.D., F.A.C.S., clinical professor of plastic surgery at Colorado University, said, "If a woman has constant neck or back pain, she should first see her doctor and follow a medical regimen. When, after two or three months, this does not alleviate the problem, she should see a plastic surgeon."

The operation is not a simple one but it's usually safe when performed by a certified plastic surgeon. There are risks with

---

* Psycho-Cybernetics, reprinted by permission of the publisher, Prentice Hall, a division of Simon & Schuster, Englewood Cliffs, NJ.

any surgery but they are reduced by closely following the physician's advice both before and after surgery. The procedure removes fat, glandular tissue, and skin, making breasts smaller, lighter, and firmer. It reduces the size of the darker skin surrounding the nipple and gives the woman better-shaped breasts in proportion to the rest of her body. A woman who had breast reduction when she was in her fifties said, "No matter how many pounds I lost, I still looked overweight. I can't describe how wonderful I feel with my lighter figure."

If a woman is obese, she must lose weight before considering this operation. Guidelines are provided on eating, drinking, smoking and taking or avoiding certain vitamins and medications. Aspirin and any anti-inflammatory agent must not be taken because they interfere with coagulation.

The cost ranges from $2,500 to $10,000, depending upon the surgical variables and the city and state where you reside. If breast reduction is medically necessary, some insurance companies pay for it with certain restrictions.

When a woman decides to go ahead with the surgery, she should adapt her schedule to the plastic surgeon's. For example, she should not ask him to change his planning or scheduling.to suit her convenience. If he operates at a certain hospital, it is inappropriate to ask him to go to another. (Believe it or not, some women do this!) Competent surgeons have established efficient routines that they know from experience yield the best results for the doctor and the patient. It is to her advantage to follow the details of his program for surgery and recovery. Her doctor will advise her about what to expect after the operation and during recuperation.

The usual at-home healing period is two weeks, then she can return to work. During the recuperation period – about two months – she wears a support system. Dr. Hoehn said, "I have found that women are more grateful for this operation than for any other in plastic surgery. It is a very satisfying procedure."

Every effort has been made to insure that the information in this chapter is current. Progress marches on and better procedures are continuing to be researched, tested and utilized.

For your particular need, the most proficient physician may or may not have the highest fees. But, authoritative advice, in the final analysis, is the least expensive way to go. It is wise to have all your questions answered. Qualified physicians will welcome them and will be pleased that you are concerned enough to ask.

# 6

# Where Is Your Hair Headed?

"Hair, like makeup, can be an
effective line hider."
—Carlotta Karlson Jacobson[1]

Unless you wear tiger skins or purple hair, the face is the focal point of your appearance with the hair acting as a flattering frame. The hair should not compete with, overpower or detract from the face.

Since regular exercise is good for the body, it is good for the hair, too. Physical activity and massaging boost circulation. They also alleviate tensions, which can be harmful to hair.

Proper maintenance becomes increasingly important as hair begins to lose elasticity, moisture and volume. Hair is not self-sustaining. Give it consistent care and conditioning with products fortified with beneficial additives. These simple one-minute routines also help:

*Brushing.* Keep it gentle not vigorous. Be especially careful with the hair bordering the forehead because it is fragile. Brush this area with a gentle touch. Using a brush with wide-spaced bristles, bend over (either standing or sitting) and brush the hair down toward the floor, stroking from the nape of the neck to the forehead. Feel the bristles grazing the scalp where the life of the hair is. This stimulates the oil glands and increases the circulation. Do not overbrush. More than 15 strokes may be too much, especially if your hair breaks

103

easily. Or, use fingers to comb through, stroking the scalp with your nails.

*Massage.* A tight scalp may suggest poor circulation. Spread fingers firmly on your head. With a circular motion, move the skin over the bone. Massage one area until it tingles then move on to the next.

*Nutrition.* Hair is made from protein and thrives on it. Protein in the following foods strengthens and promotes growth: Fish, eggs and dairy products; grains ex. oatmeal, rye, brown rice; legumes ex. garbanzos, peas, limas; nuts and seeds ex. sesame, almonds, cashews; green leaves i.e. parsley, collards, spinach, broccoli, cauliflower; potatoes and many others.[2] B complex vitamins with biotin and riboflavin are essential for the body's utilization of protein. Excessive sugar, salt, alcohol and caffeine are not good for the hair.[3]

Rather than overload your body with supplements, check with a nutritionist to see what you need. Vitamins and minerals cannot correct poor hair conditions caused by underlying medical problems.

## Maintenance

Oil treatments and weekly conditioning with products that contain healthy boosters restores the natural moisture level. These processes are especially important for permed, frosted or bleached hair.

Buy products for your type of hair (dry, normal, oily) and condition (permed, frosted or treated). Frequently, hair care companies use natural ingredients that come from the sea, plants, fruits and flower extracts. If you worry about multi-syllabic chemicals, investigate products that have ingredients you recognize.

Ask your hairdresser what products you should use for your type of hair. Most women over 50 need a conditioner after shampooing. Does she use one on your hair?

*Cleansing.* Because the scalp produces less and less oil, shampooing once a week is sufficient for most of us. Even hair that has not been permed or bleached is damaged by harsh shampoos or soaps. Protein-rich shampoos protect the hair and keep it from looking drab. Regular shampoo is poison for color-treated hair because it flattens the color. To keep hair color fresh and true, use a color-enhancing shampoo. For perms, look for one specifically for chemically treated hair. Otherwise, a shampoo can relax the curl.

Before shampooing, massage your scalp to circulate the oil sitting on the skin. Improper shampooing is often the cause of problem hair. This method will keep you from botching it:

1.  Don't punish your hair with hot water! Wet hair thoroughly with warm water. Pour the shampoo into your palm and rub hands together. Massage it into the scalp, moving the skin over the bone as you cleanse. If you need more lather, add a little water rather than more shampoo.

2.  Rinsing is very important. Rinse three to four times longer than you shampoo to remove every trace of lather. Cool water for the final rinse flattens the shaft, promotes shine and invigorates. Apply a conditioner.

3.  Be gentle with wet hair. Pat dry to prevent breakage.

*Conditioning.* Doing it after shampooing with a protein-packed product restores elasticity, moisture and oils. This is essential for us. Because of stress, chemical processing, and environmental pollutants, the formulas for conditioners are now beneficial to both hair and scalp. The labeling on the product describes its purpose. Therapeutic conditioners, created for fragile African-American hair that breaks easily, are available. Grocery stores, drugstores and beauty salons have excellent conditioners. Some are pH balanced, 100 percent oil free, and dermatologist tested. Extra mild conditioners are available when frequent shampooing is necessary. The functions of conditioners are to:

- Replenish moisture
- Protect from damaging elements, such as the weather and sun
- Repair frequently styled, permed or color treated hair
- Add body to limp, fine or thinning hair
- Increase shine, vitality and manageability without relaxing curl
- Neutralize unwanted yellowing from grey and white hair.

Don't over-condition! Too much of a good thing is just that, too much. Read the directions. A lot can be learned by talking with knowledgeable consultants in salons and beauty schools.

*Hair Spray, Mousse and Gels.* Use alcohol-free products that do not dull or dry. Mousse has the lightest hold; spray has light, medium and strong hold; and gels the strongest. Use gel on damp, not soaked, hair where you need extra body or hold. Too much of either product weighs hair down.

Hair sprays can provide moisture, shine, and sunscreen protection. Use one with medium or strong hold for styling. Simply brush; spray; lift, smooth or separate with a hair pick; spray again to set. You have another choice if you have lots of hair and want a free-flowing feel: Shake your head while spraying your hair.

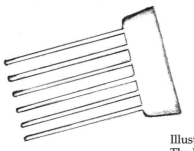

Illustration 18
The Useful Hair Pick

*Dull-looking Hair.* Shine lessens because the sebaceous glands produce less and less oil. Proper rinsing is one part of improvement. A lemon juice rinse brightens, but is also drying. Conditioners, hair sprays, and shampoos have ingredients that add luster. Twice a month treat your hair to a deep penetrating moisturizing conditioner. Rub conditioner between your palms and then on your hair working from ends toward the scalp. Leave it on 20 minutes before rinsing.

Warm oil treatments are excellent all-around conditioners that improve sheen. You can do it yourself with this recipe:

Heat either olive, sesame or coconut oil to warm.
Distribute evenly with fingers from scalp to the ends.
Cover with thin plastic, then wrap a towel that has been saturated in hot water and rung out over the plastic, or, sit under a hair dryer.
Wait for 15 minutes, then shampoo, lathering twice and rinse thoroughly.

---

Dry hair? Try an overnight olive oil "bath." Pour on enough oil to saturate and finger comb from roots to tips. Sleep on a towel-covered pillow. In the morning shampoo and rinse well to remove all oil.

---

*Fine and Thin Hair.* Fine hair refers to the diameter of each strand that is so small the hair is limp. Thin refers to the number of hairs, which usually decreases with age. If your hair is thinning, you may wish to consult a dermatologist. Rogaine, the brand name for minoxidil and approved by the FDA, is an over-the-counter drug that helps some people.

Massaging to increase circulation, proper shampooing, conditioning and products specifically labeled for fine and thin hair help. Products with body-building ingredients like panthenol and biotin (vitamin B factors), collagen (a form of protein), and magnesium add volume.

Look for products that have "volume" or "volumizing" in the labeling. Aveda, Aussie, Redken and Nexxus have volumizing shampoo. Or, try Bumble & Bumble Hair Thickening Spray. You want a spray that gives shine and medium hold, one that doesn't weight hair down. Read the label. Some hair dryers have volumizing attachments like the Braun Super Volume Hair Dryer.

Permanent coloring and fine-hair body perms thicken shafts and make hair easier to manage. Tight curly perms clump strands together, making the hair look less full. A chic short cut with texturizing – a clipping technique that increases volume – does not weigh fine hair down the way a longer length does.

## Perming

Better products are constantly coming on the market. Your hairdresser should use the best ones for your type of hair. Or, do it yourself and carefully read the labeling and directions. Too much chemical processing will dry and dull hair and can create problems. If you color, perm only if it is absolutely necessary. When it is, perm first and wait at least two to three weeks before coloring. Think in terms of a body wave for extra fullness no more than twice a year, preferably in the spring and fall. If you only need a touch-up for a place that needs more curl or wave, then, get a spot perm.

For women who are disabled, the wash and dry tight perm is best. It requires minimal care with just a daily soft brushing or run-through with the fingers.

## No-Perm Curling

Women who want soft curl but not overnight curlers opt for the a steam-roller curling system, found in drugstores and beauty supply stores. It takes about 15 minutes to set and curl. Be sure to get small rollers if your hair is short. Women with straight-as-a-pin hair use it successfully, saving time and money. Flowing and wavy is more youthful than tight and kinky. You can also use the curling iron to bend, curl or wave stubborn hair.

## Coloring Erases Years

Both skin and hair lose color. The combination of a pale complexion with greying hair is not a winning combo, so add color – blond, a soft red or brown. Coloring the hair gives more vitality to the face and lifts the spirits.

A friend was depressed about her white hair because she didn't feel as old as she looked. She had it colored a natural-looking golden blond and was amazed at how much better she looked *and felt*. At a family reunion, her relatives said she seemed to be the only one who wasn't getting older!

Grey or white hair on women whose skin has yellow undertones, such as the one mentioned above, look older and are happy with a color change. When they have blue or pink undertones, white and silver grey hair can be very attractive, providing it is not dull or yellowish. If it is, look for shampoos that remove the brassiness and brighten the white or grey. Drugstores and salons carry these.

Select hair coloring according to the undertones of the skin. (See page 10 for specific information on undertones.)

| Blue/Pink Undertones (cool) | Yellow Undertones (warm) |
| --- | --- |
| Ash blond | Golden blond |
| Silver grey and white | Flaxen blond |
| Ash brown | Golden brown |
| Blue black and blue brown | Red brown |

If your skin is fair, avoid dark shades. They magnify lines and wrinkles. You may choose an all-over or partial coloring. Highlighting the hair around the temples uplifts droopy eyes and minimizes facial lines. An added bonus is that bleaching swells the shaft and gives it more body and manageability.

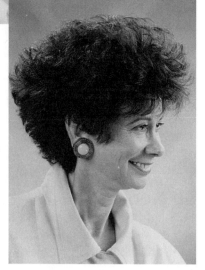

"The woman, not the years,
is the focus of my designs."
Hair and Makeup by Designer
Angela Grandinetti, Hair Cartel in Denver, CO

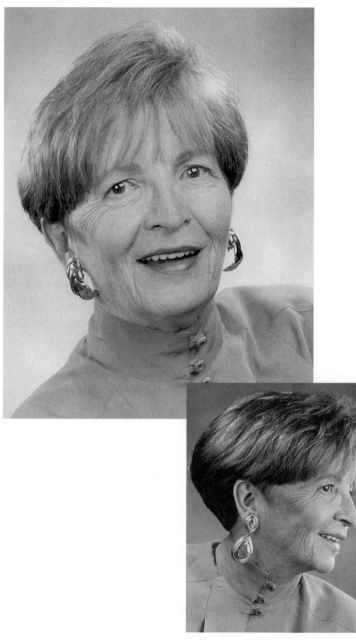

Hair and Makeup by Designer
Angela Grandinetti, Hair Cartel in Denver, CO

Color shampoos and mousses add color that lasts from shampoo to shampoo. The effectiveness of these products depends upon the porosity of the hair, its ability to absorb the color. Chemically treated hair – permed or bleached – has more porosity. These processes swell the hair shaft and give it more body and manageability. Women who have colored their hair for years still maintain healthy-looking tresses. They nourish the hair on the outside, the body on the inside and keep the body physically activated.

> Look good coming and going. Fuss with
> the front AND back of your hair.

## *"How Do I Find a Good Hairdresser?"*

At this time, hair salons have shown little ingenuity in creating unique and individual styles for the modern 50-plus woman. As we get older, they have one generic hairdo – short, teased or fluffed all over, with a forehead curl here or there. This is okay for some, but for all of us? On the other hand, have we been content with the same old style thinking the smart look is not for us? Well, it is. A new, chic, youthful hairstyle is wonderful for the morale.

To find a good stylist, ask women – even strangers whose hairstyle you admire – who does their hair. Call the manager of a beauty school. They get lots of feed-back. Watch newspaper ads, or consult the Yellow Pages and telephone several in locations convenient to you. Make a short list of questions such as:

"Do you have an operator that is especially good at styling hair for women over 50? I would like something different and more up-to-date."

If they hem and haw over this question, cross them off your list. The way they respond tells a lot. You do not want a hairdresser who has out-dated misconceptions of how a modern woman over 50 should look.

"My hair is greying and I want a change. Do you have an experienced colorist who can advise me as to whether I should color my hair?"

If you want coloring, cutting and styling, speak to the manager of the shop to find out who is proficient in all three.

## How to Work with a Hairdresser to Get the Best Results

How many times have you come home from the hairdresser and recombed your hair? Seldom do stylists consider the overall appearance and personality before they take the scissors. Tell them about your lifestyle and show pictures of hairstyles you like. This is more effective than groping for words to describe something you may not be too sure of.

Scan magazines and fashion brochures for hairstyles you would like to imitate. Collect pictures, the age of the woman in the photo is unimportant, only the hair. Don't get bogged down in analyzing whether a style will look right on you. That comes during your consultation with the hairdresser when you discuss whether a certain style or variation would be best.

The contours of the head, face, figure, and your personality determine the most flattering style. When you are discussing a new hairstyle, keep in mind the following:

- If your nose is prominent, you need fullness at the back of the head.
- Bangs balance a high or broad forehead and focus attention on the eyes.
- Wear short hair for a short neck and longer hair for the longer neck.
- Hair on sides should have a combined width no greater than the width of your face.

- The height of your hair should not exceed the length of your forehead.
- If you are large-boned, tall or broad shouldered, your hair should be full, not skimpy, to balance the proportion of your figure. Conversely, if you are petite, your style needs to be closer to the head and slightly higher on top.

- Usually, the athletic woman may not care to look like a *grande dame de Paris*. She is more comfortable with an easy-to-care-for style as is the very busy woman.

Hair that is too long, too curly, too bouffant, too set is too old-looking. The lines of our hairstyles require movement. A gamin-type haircut – close-cropped in back, straight at the sides with straight bangs – may have been charming for years, but when facial lines and shadows become noticeable, this cut draws attention to them. The severity of extremes on most of us, such as the all-over upsweeps, emphasizes facial lines. So does hair that is teased too high or too wide at the sides or cut too short. Instead, choose a cut that flows and moves.

Although short hair is a popular choice, it is not for everyone. Some women will never wear it. A woman I knew had an abundance of shiny, snow-white, softly waving hair. She wore it shoulder-length. This style was perfect for her slim figure, long throat and peppy personality.

Change is good and sometimes scary. That may be why we stick with one style. Many times we hesitate to voice our ideas or fears and then wonder why we don't get what we want. Talk them over with your hairdresser, so he/she understands you better. Treat the stylist as an interested friend. Then, don't snooze off. Pay attention to what is done. If they start to tease (back comb) and you don't want teasing, say so. It can easily be smoothed out. Hairdressers tease the hair to give it more body. Ask if they have a body-building shampoo and conditioner. If they don't, bring your own.

If you are unhappy with the results, talk about it before getting out of the chair. Feel comfortable saying, "I don't like the way my hair curls here" or "Can the color be softened?" or "Can you give me more height here?" Be specific. Don't be a cranky critic, establish an intelligent relationship through honest dialogues.

Conscientious hairstylists take pleasure in a beautifully styled hairdo that becomes the client. It's good advertising for them. When you are puzzled about how to get the same results after you leave their skillful fingers, ask how you can work with your hair between appointments. A contented customer is a valuable asset, and so is a good hairdresser.

## *Shaping*

Great hairdos start with great cuts. When the cut still brushes into shape after three weeks, you know you've had a good one. Hair looks best and is easiest to care for when it is trimmed every four to six weeks.

Hair is shaped to balance and harmonize with the shape of the face. To do this, the hair should fluff out at the narrowest part of the face and be closer to the head at the widest. The following guidelines illustrate how to shape the hair according to the shape of the face:

*Oval Face.* Best bet is simple, a little wavy and in proportion to the face. Hair looks best when it flows away from the face. Off-center styles break the regular lines. Fullness at the sides can make the face seem long and narrow. Wispy bangs draw attention to the eyes and give the face more contour.

*Thin Face.* Curls, fullness and highlights at the sides make this face appear wider and more oval. (See Illustration 19.)

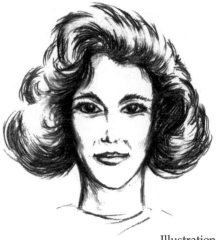

Illustration 19
Hair Shape for a Thin Face

*Triangular Face.* Style hair close to the head at the widest part of the face and full at the narrowest part. Direct waves and curls towards the narrowest part. There are two kinds of this type:

1. *Narrow at forehead, cheeks and brows, wider at chin and jaw-bone, pear-shaped.* A center or low side part adds width to the brows. At the forehead, have bangs that are soft and non-uniform, maybe flaring out at each side. Pulling the hair back from the forehead and temples is a no-no. Cut hair to earlobes or slightly above.

2. *Inverted triangle, heart-shaped.* Broad forehead with narrow jawline: Wear hair close to the head and fuller from the eyes to chin, neck and shoulder areas. Try a high side part and waves or wispy bangs. Do not cut hair shorter than the bottoms of the earlobes. (See Illustration 20.)

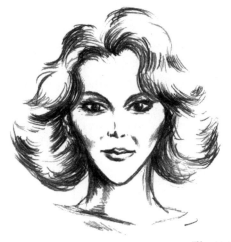

Illustration 20
Hair Shape for
Inverted Triangle Face

*Narrow Chin.* Wear hair a little below the ears with full-ness or curls at jawline to balance receding jaw or pointed chin. (See Illustration 21.)

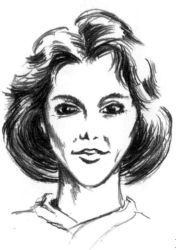

Illustration 21
Hair Shape for
Narrow Chin

*Round Face.* Cut the hair to the bottom of the earlobes with height and fullness on top and a high side part. Soft waves or curls toward the center of the crown gives needed height. Add highlights at the top. Sides should wave back and up. Longer hair should surround the face with curls/waves concentrating on the jaw, neck or shoulder area. Side-swept bangs lengthen.

*Square Face.* An off-center part or soft, curly bangs swept to the sides soften the wide brow. Brush sides toward the face with volume above the forehead and gentle waves flowing back. Keep the hair styled close to the head at wide cheekbones. Straight hair and straight bangs do not flatter.

*Wide Chin or Jaw.* Keep hair short. Use soft curls/waves and fullness at the sides to balance out the strong chin.

*Long Face.* Wear a medium length, full on the sides. Straight hanging hair makes your face seem drawn. Break the long line with curls and layering, and soft bangs for the high forehead. (See Illustration 22.)

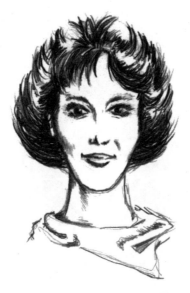

Illustration 22
Hair Shape for Long Face

*Low Forehead.* Avoid bangs; use soft fullness above the forehead and at the crown to lengthen the forehead. Add highlights around the front of the hairline.

> A quick and easy hairfix:
> Brush hair head-down and spray if you
> want more fullness. When you raise your
> head, smooth, shape and spray to set.

## Wigs

"I can't think of any negatives about them!" enthused a wig-wearing woman. "They feel comfortable, look as good as my real hair and require minimal styling. They're fantastic!" and she wear wigs at least 40 hours every week. After discovering she had cancer and, before chemotherapy began, she bought two wigs, one the same color as her hair and the other a mix of lighter shades. Many people told her they couldn't see any difference between the wigs and her real hair. At the end of the treatments, her hair grew back as thick and beautiful as ever.

Another friend developed a disease of the scalp resulting in hair loss that was caused, she said, by too much perming and coloring. Under the care of a dermatologist, she faithfully followed a remedial routine, and her hair grew back almost as full as before. But in the meantime, she loved wearing wigs. When she wore one that was golden brown, people told her she looked years younger. She enhanced it with more naturalness by combing some of the white hair around her forehead into the wig hair.

Both women were not conscious of having a wig on because they are ultra lightweight. The second woman said the money she saved in shampoos, sets and cuts for two months equaled the cost of one wig. Working women buy them for convenience, others for the fun of it.

Here are some tips:

- When you shop for a wig, take a friend along (a must) and try to find an understanding, knowledgeable salesperson either in a wig shop or department store, who takes a personal interest in you, not just in making a sale.

- Color is very important. The right color beautifies your complexion and brings out the color of your eyes. Check it out in daylight because store light can be deceptive.

- Expect some frustration in finding the right one. Try on several. Don't buy on the first visit because the trying-on process is tiring. Come back when you are refreshed and have had time to think about it.

- Go without a wig as often as you can. Air is important to the growth of new hair.

- Women who have lost or are losing their hair should acquire two or three turbans or fashionable caps so they will feel comfortable during their wig-free time.

Wigs are full of promise and a wonderful solution for women who are devastated by the loss of hair, who want the convenience and time-saving advantages, or who are in the mood for an exciting change.

> Every hair does not have to be in place!
> In fact, the slightly blown-away
> look is great for us.

# 7

# Fashion for
# Your Figure

Modern women who are past midlife are not waiting for life to roll by. They are grabbing and squeezing it for all it's worth. Regardless of your age, size or skin color, you can have a smart, attractive head-to-toe image. To create it, positive thinking, planning, desire and a can-do attitude are required. Vitality in appearance results from vitality in thinking. This is not a complicated process. Simplicity combined with color is a winning combination.

No body is perfect! And no amount of exercise or dieting alters your basic body structure. When weight change is impossible, accept the way you are. Spend your energy drawing attention to your best features and de-emphasizing the not-so-good ones. The following elements of design are basic to enhancement and camouflage:

*Line* – Vertical lines in the cut of the garment and the use of color add length to your figure. Horizontal lines in the cut and print of the fabric add width.

*Color* – Smart use of color creates optical illusions, making the figure appear bigger, thinner or better than it is. Monochromatic outfits and one-color apparel slenderize. Use light and bright colors to accent your best features. Darker or neutral ones play down the pounds or minimize unattractive proportions. White gives a bigger look. If worn around the face, it can drain color from the complexion, showing up lines and shadows.

*Textures of Fabrics* – Fuzzy, tweedy and shiny fabrics seem to add weight to the figure. Shiny fabrics and soft textures around the throat are becoming to the face. Smooth, fine knits accent contours more than those with a nap, such as bouclés or nubby weaves. Contrasting textures, such as a cashmere sweater with a silk skirt, smack of sublime style. Natural materials – cotton, wool, silk, linen – have an easy-to-wear simplicity appropriate for all seasons. Resiliency – the ability of a fabric to resist wrinkling – is often improved when natural fibers are combined with synthetics.

## Body Types

Practically every body type can be attractive when it is adorned in clothing that camouflages the negatives and accentuates the positives. Check out the type(s) that fit your figure. Most of us fit into two or more categories. When you know how to fit your figure according to color, line and fabric, shopping is easier and clothing is comfortable and enjoyable to wear.

*Evenly Proportioned/Average Height.* With balanced proportions, you can wear color a variety of ways. Bright colors enlarge. If this is not a problem, use them on your best features. Analyze your figure. Use vertical lines where you want to slenderize and horizontals where you need fullness or width.

*Triangle/Narrow at Shoulders with Larger Hips and Legs.* To de-emphasize large hips choose jackets that are hip- or thigh-length. Keep bright colors and interest items above the waist; wear subdued or darker shades below. Draw attention up with ropes of beads or shiny metals.

The additional width of shoulder pads trim the waist and hip line, improving upper body proportions. Padding should conform to the bone structure with subtle extension. (See Illustration 23.) Padding that is obviously bulky or extends far

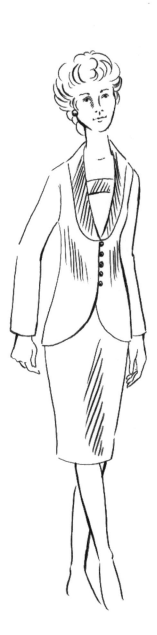
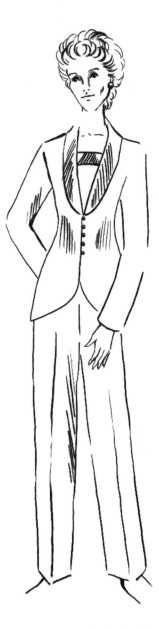

Illustration 23
Shoulder pads
narrow the waist
and hip lines

beyond the shoulder line overpowers upper body proportions, especially if you are under 5'4". A chemise with built-in pads, makes them less obvious than some garments that have pads attached. You can also get clip-on pads that create a curvy or square shape.

Super-long, super-sleek separates create a slimmer look, as do man-tailored slacks with room at the top. Be careful with pleats. If the silhouette is too baggy, you'll look hippy. Inverted pleats are best. (See Illustration 24.) Let trousers fall straight with no flap around the ankles. If you are 5'4" or less, a cuffless hem gives a longer line. Mid-calf pants balance wide hips.

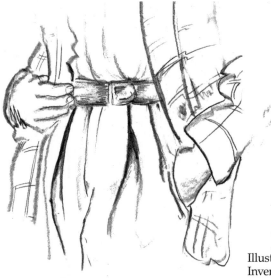

Illustration 24
Inverted Pleats

Use simple, slightly flared skirts, fitting but not tight at the hips. Long narrow skirts in solid colors with matching hose and shoes are slimming. Gathered skirts add pounds to the hips. Wear skirts that flair below the hips, and sweaters, shirts and overblouses that go down to the point where the flair begins. Patch pockets on the hips and wide belts make hips look wider. Narrow belts are appropriate.

*Inverted Triangle/Wide Shoulders, Narrow Torso.* Use subdued colors on upper body with a dark tailored jacket and matching skirt or slacks. Color on pockets at hipline add width to the narrow part of your figure. Bright colors are best worn below the waist. Man-style shirts in crisp fabrics and oversize sweaters and dresses without shoulder pads will not give a top heavy look. Be wary of shoulder pads that do. Skirts with pleats or flair balance the wide shoulder line.

*Plump or Overweight.* Vertical panels of color from shoulders to hemline slenderize, such as a two-toned suit with one side of the jacket in a neutral, the other side, a darker color. (See Illustration 25.) Stay away from horizontal lines and plaids. Use bright colors for small accents.

Rather than contrasting colors, such as a white blouse with black slacks, try monochromatic combinations, e.g., a pearl grey blouse with slacks or skirt in a darker grey or vice versa, depending upon the proportions of your figure. One-color and monochromatic dressing for the large woman creates the illusion of tall and trim. Fake out fat with long uninterrupted lines – vertical ribbing and generously cut cable knits or cardigans with a plunging neckline.

Go for oversized sweaters, overblouses and tunics with simple skirts or straight-leg (no flair) slacks. Acid-wash jeans add pounds, as do dirndl skirts. Skirts with deep pleats or gathers make even a slim figure look chunky. Depending on your height, keep hems just below knees or mid-calf. If you are petite, let hems be no longer than mid-knee. Shoulder pads square the upper body and give the illusion of narrowing the hip area – an important factor for this body type.

Wear only your most flattering colors, and fabrics that move with simple, fluid lines, such as fine knits, lightweight cottons, soft cashmeres and silks. Try linens, crisp cottons and gabardines if they fit your style and slenderize. Tight fits outline bulges.

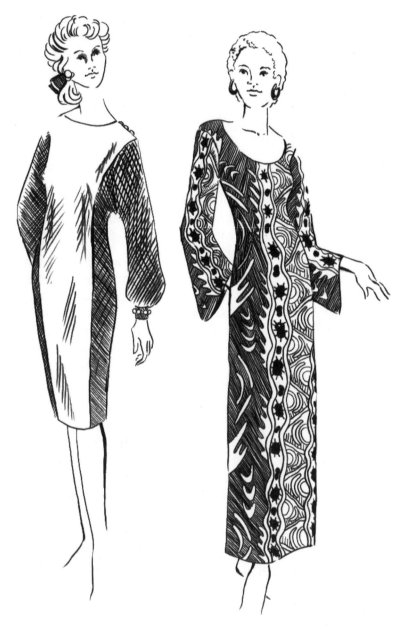

Illustration 25
Vertical lines in cut, color
and design slenderize.

*Too Thin.* A woman in a seminar asked, "Everyone talks about women who are too fat, what about people like me who are too thin?"

They can use the opposite of everything described for the plump figure, adapting the dressmaking lines and color design to your height and the proportions of your figure. Prints with bold horizontal lines, bright and contrasting colors, fitted jackets, textured fabrics, big knits, full, flowing skirts, and pleated slacks can all be in your closet. Don't forget shoulder pads to tailor the torso.

*5'7" and Over.* Wear contrasting colors, top and bottom. Interrupt one-color outfits with a contrasting color in belt or peplin. Use color interest in large handbags, jewelry and accessories. Horizontal lines and plaids balance with your height. Wear jackets that come below the hipline. For slacks, pleats are fine if you are not too hippy, and so are cuffs. For large hips, slacks with straight lines look best.

Summer-cool loose, full pants or skirts are lovely on the taller figure if they are cut in body-conscious ways and/or sharpened with graphic prints.

*Under 5'7" – Petite.* Try vertical lines in the color, print and the cut of apparel. No belts unless you wear them under a jacket or vest. Belts of the same fabric or color do not interrupt the one-color line as much as those in a contrasting color. Hems are around mid-knee or floor length. If you are long-waisted, wear jackets or sweaters that come to the hips or a little below. Long narrow pants without cuffs make you look taller and slimmer. All-season gabardine slacks are a good bet. Wear a tunic or sweater to cover. Full tops complements slim pants.

## Camouflaging Figure Challenges

The basics are:

- To de-emphasize, use dark or neutral colors.
- To slenderize, wear vertical lines in color and style.

Monochromatic dressing elongates your figure. (See Illustration 25.)

■ To widen or add pounds, use horizontal lines in the cut of the garment and in color with light, bright shades.

*Sagging Bosoms.* Nothing ages a figure more than breasts that droop. A supportive bra restores a youthful figure line and allows clothing to hang better. An uplifted bosom corrects the matronly look. Bras with wider straps do not dig into the shoulders. You can also purchase velcro attachments (found in the notions departments) that fit onto the straps.

When I mentioned improving the bust line in a *Glamour for Grandmas* class, the women couldn't resist covertly scanning everyone's chest. Suddenly, one woman blurted out, "My, yours sure look good!" We followed her gaze to Ann, whose trim sweater revealed a teen-like bustline. "Well, they should," she said with a note of satisfaction. "This is a $500 bra!" To answer our astonishment, she explained she had had a double mastectomy. "Ever since I was in high school, my pendulous breasts were burdensome and embarrassing. Now I can look the way I want to!"

*Full Bust.* Get a brassiere that has diagonal seaming rather than horizontal in the cup. When a woman has breasts that are different in size, and many of us do, this cut does a better job of equalizing them. Playtex and Maidenform sell them. If support is more important than lift, call Decent Exposures 1-800-524-4949 for their free catalogue. They have fit every size and shape from 28AAA to 58H.

Use shallow V-necks, the shawl neckline, or convertible and open collars at the throat. Cardigan and Chanel jackets, the A-line shift and shirt-waist styles are good. No gaping button fronts! Remedy by inserting gussets under the arms. Quilted, embroidered, beaded, sequined or studded details in the shoulder area or a large colorful broach/pin on this upper line draws the gaze up.

For workouts and body-jerking activities like Jazzercise, fast walking and some sports, the sports bra offers comfort and controls bounce. One style fits and flatters with a front opening. They come in different colors and are great for casual wear when you are carefree about shape.

*Heavy Upper Arms.* No strapless, sleeveless fashions or skinny knit sleeves. Opt for full-cut sleeves, such as dolmen or kimono. Sleeves can be rolled to the elbows but keep them loose-fitting.

> Good fashion sense whispers that
> covering jiggly or skinny arms
> gives the better look.

*Stooped Shoulders/Rounded Back.* Shirt collars are better than jewel necklines. Big soft scarves flatter, not narrow skimpy ones. Avoid fabrics that cling to the upper body. Go for fabrics with texture – bouclé, fuzzy, nubby – rather than flat knits. Allow blouses and jackets to be full across the back of the throat and have enough body to hang straight. No belts. You can visualize how a fitted garment accentuates contours. The same applies to coats.

For an additional lift, brush hair away from your face and throat. In the back, cultivate a soft, swept-up short coiffure. Avoid straight, severe cuts.

*No Waistline.* Don't wear belts on anything, not even coats. Wear straight lines, shoulders to hips, and no one will know your waist size. An exceptionally well-groomed woman I know is 5'2", slightly over-weight with no waist, yet people often compliment her on what she wears and ask her advice. She honed her skill to camouflage an imperfect figure so effectively that the "limitations" were never obvious. She had no special training, but thoughtfully observed, compared, analyzed and enjoyed designing and redesigning her clothes.

### *Plump Mid-Section.*

1.  Use darker shades below the waist and no shiny fabrics.

2.  One-color outfits without belts minimize. Wear belts under vests or jackets.

3.  Avoid fitted clothing and clingy fabrics, nothing too tight or revealing.

4.  No fuss in front – no pleats, pockets, ornate buttons to detract from a streamlined look.

5.  Shirt-waist dresses with straight lines, fullness above and below the waist flatter.

6.  Roomy, not sloppy, jackets, overblouses, and long sweaters conceal. If you are tall or long-waisted, these garments may come to or below the hip line. Get vested! Vests in all colors and fabrics hide a thick waist.

7.  Color accents around the throat and shoulders draw attention away from the torso, as do interesting necklines designed with scarves or jewelry.

8.  Bolder shoulders with pads take inches off the midsection and eliminate the egg-shaped look.

9.  Be wary of gathered or full-pleated skirts, especially if you are under 5'3". They make even a slim figure appear chunky.

10. Never buy pocketless side-zip jeans. The zipper bulge is too prominent. Tight jeans draw attention to figure lines. They better be good! Otherwise, keep them loose-fitting with front pleats or a V-seamed front yoke. (See Illustration 26.)

11. Girdles are not what they used to be. Lightweight and tissue-thin, they are machine washable, spun in spandex and nylon, and provide good control without discomfort. Some have a high waist to smooth out a mid-section roll. The all-in-one combination of bra and girdle is a comfortable and firming alternative.

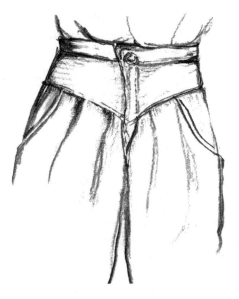

Illustration 26
The V-seamed Yoke

*Extra Weight on Outer Thighs.* You have choices. For slacks, sleek, straight, long lines are slimming. Let them taper to the ankles, no flapping hems unless you are over 5'5". If hips are wide, too much taper creates a balloon effect. Full-cut pants and looser legs create a flattering roomy (not baggy) look. Choose the one that looks best on your figure. Pleats in slacks should not be too full. Eliminate bulges by having pockets in front not on sides. Stretchy fabrics exaggerate contours, as do mottled acid-wash jeans. A vertical row of buttons, dark colors such as black, navy and charcoal – uniform color – are as slenderizing as a diet. A-line or wrap skirts emphasize body length and hide thighs.

*Broad Hips.* The hem of a jacket should be above the widest part of the hips if you are short waisted. The longer jacket provides coverup. One-color outfits and darker tones below the waistline will de-emphasize. Front pockets on trousers draw attention to this area. Slash pockets are better.

*Heavy Legs.* Slacks with deep pleats fall smoothly over heavy legs. Clinging fabrics add pounds and draw attention to bulges. Legs look longer and thinner when hosiery is toned to skirt and shoes. Darker shades, such as black, do it better than light ones. Higher heels always make legs look thinner.

***Thin Legs.*** Pleated slacks camouflage. Light colored hose fill out thin legs. Slim skirts that come to or below the knee cover the thinner thigh while showing off the shapeliest part of your legs, the calves. Avoid A-line and full skirts, and bulky fabrics like tweedy wools and wide-wale corduroys that make thin legs look stick-like. If you want a long, full skirt, select one in a soft, flowing fabric – rayons, silks, cotton knits – with flat or low-heeled shoes.

***The Hemline.*** Generally, hemlines should be worn at the knee or lower, depending on your height. Be sure the hem does not stop at the heaviest part of your legs. Wear it either higher or lower. If weight has shifted from back to front, have your skirts re-hemmed to be sure they fall evenly all the way around.

***Sports Attire.*** Doctors and experts continually emphasize the importance of a regular program of physical activity. Let your sports clothing be fun to wear and comfortable. Check out the stretchy support shorts in the lingerie department. They are nifty under shorts, slacks and long cotton shirts. Elasticized leggings also make legs look good under shorts and long T's. We mentioned the sports bra in this chapter under "Full Bust." Some department stores have a "plus size" sportswear department.

## *Do's*

Simplicity defines ageless.

Wear fun colors and bold, light-hearted prints.

Show off pretty legs in modestly slit skirts with mid-knee hems especially if you are petite.

Faded jeans with a long, soft sweater and shiny black loafers or boots always look smart, so do tailored slacks.

## Don'ts

The vamp look.

Short shorts and miniskirts.

Tight, cheap T-shirts.

Baggy pants, sloppy tops and too long skirts.

Deliberately trying to 'do' young is frustrating. Find what's becoming as your body changes and compliment the good features; cover the not-so-good ones. Your best style is determined by what is lifestyle- and body-appropriate, not by what is age-appropriate.

Make a checklist of the flattering fashion factors for your figure and keep them in mind when you shop. It simplifies selection. Women over 50 have graduated beyond fads, miniskirts and bikinis. Still, they are fun-loving and feel years and sometimes decades younger than their age. They want their timeless image to reflect that feeling with wardrobe selections tailored to their interests and activities. They want fabric textures and styles lines that feel good on the body – apparel that is adaptable to different climatic conditions indoors as well as out, easy to pack and practical for travel.

## Shop Like a Professional

- Don't shop when you're hurried, hungry, tired or moody. You'll buy on impulse just to get relief.

- If your budget is tight and a special occasion is coming up, you may not need a new head-to-toe outfit. Instead, why not get a new accessory or two?

- Go slow on sales. They are not always bargains and markdowns can be lousy buys. Ask yourself: If I had the money, would I buy it at full price? If yes, then, it's a find.

- Don't buy anything too tight. You may not lose five pounds!

- Don't buy slacks without the sit/bend test or you may have to stand up in them.

- New technology is improving the quality of synthetics. Good polyester charmeuse beats poor quality silk. Search for blends in which the natural fiber dominates.

- Best buys are made of year-round fabrics such as silk, viscose, wool and cotton. Versatile blends with natural fibers are cool in summer and can be layered in winter.

- Two-color outfits never fail. If a third color comes into play, make it a neutral, such as white, grey, beige, brown, navy or black.

- Judge clothes by the fit, not the size on the tag. Standard sizes change from company to company and even within a company which may re-evaluate the sizing. Check out the front, back *and side view*. Try on as many sizes as necessary to get a good fit. Sometimes, the cut of the garment, not the size, poses a problem.

- Before you buy, ask yourself: Do I have the body for this fashion? Does it go with at least two other items I already have? Think simplicity, ease, comfort, color.

- Look for details that indicate quality: fine-tooth zippers in neat plackets; bound buttonholes; shoulder pads that follow the lines of your body, neither too full nor too extended.

- Don't let sales people seduce you into compromising your taste.

- Discount fashion stores and near-new shops have some excellent merchandise at big savings.

- For the small figure, check out the boy's departments for sweats and shirts, and the girl's juniors for colorful, trendy styles. The men's departments have nifty shirts and sweaters.

- Avoid feeling indebted to helpful salespeople. Just because they looked for your size in the stock room, you don't have to buy it.

- P.T. Barnum said there's a sucker born every minute. Don't be taken in by these classic come-ons:

  "You'll just have to buy that, it's you."
  "It's a different style, but you'll get used to it."
  "Oh, you can easily alter that."
  "It's the only one left in stock. I just can't keep them on the rack."
  "It looks great on you, and I wouldn't say that to everyone."

You are more important than your clothing. What you wear reflects your individuality and should not detract from the person you are. Color and design, and fun and comfort are equally important. The ultimate test is, does it make you feel happy and confident?

# 8

## Hands

...think of your nails as your
BEST accessory, like a beautiful
ring, bracelet or scarf."
—Patricia Bozic[1]

Hands are always on display and are expressive. Whether they are wrinkled, spotted, veiny, or scarred, they look 100 percent better and younger when lubricated daily, manicured *and polished*. With careful conditioning, the appearance of hands and nails improves in three to four weeks.

Adrien Arpel[2] suggests soaking hands in warm olive oil for a few minutes to soften the skin and strengthen the nails. For comfort and smoothness, cleanse hands with your facial cleanser, then use a facial mask on your hands and fingers. After rinsing, massage them with an emollient cream or oil. Starting at the finger tips, as though you were putting on kid gloves, rub down each finger from tip to joint, then from joints to wrist and last, the palms. It only takes a few minutes to do a lot of good. They deserve this attention. Think of all the work they have done and will do for you.

> If you have to put your hands in water,
> add a couple tablespoons
> of vinegar to counteract dryness.

## Easy Exercise for Flexibility

A one-minute daily routine invigorates, relieves stiffness, adds flexibility and grace.

- Tightly clench fists, then splay fingers, stretching them out till you feel the stretch from palm to finger tips.

- Clench and stretch fingers five to eight times.

## Spots, Scars or Vitiligo

**Laser Treatments.** A board-certified plastic surgeon or dermatologist who specializes in the laser process for surface conditions performs these treatments on an outpatient basis. They painlessly and harmlessly remove age spots. This does not prevent new spots from appearing.

**Cosmetic Correctives.** Covermark and Dermablend are available in department stores and drugstores. They come in different shades and are natural-looking, inexpensive cover-ups.[3]

**Self-Tanning Products.** These lotions and sprays stain the skin, blending in with discolorations. Finding the color that goes with your skin may be tricky because some products have too much orange. Follow the directions. Best time to apply is after a shower or bath when the skin is warm and moist. Massage in with a circular motion. To prevent staining the fingers, wash them immediately after application. Color appears after a couple hours and stays on two to three days. It fades when exposed to water.

Manicure and polish nails with a stunning shade. Do this plus one of the three above, and your hands will look better than you ever believed possible.

## Fingernails

It is essential to healthy nails to eat foods rich in protein, fats, minerals, carbohydrates and iron. Those essentials are found in fish, liver, oats, oranges, cauliflower, dried beans, leafy greens, vitamins B biotin and B12, C, D, E, and calcium with magnesium. Liver extract tablets have nutrients and other trace minerals that may help nails, as well as hair and teeth. Elimination of toxins and good circulation are important.

Nails respond quickly to care, but nail abuse takes longer to correct. Hardeners, primers, base coats and top coats help to prevent breakage. Look for nail products that have no formaldehyde and toluene, such as the Lorik and Bareille nail systems. The acetone in polish remover is drying. Use a non-acetone remover with moisturizing properties.

Polish reinforces, enabling nails to grow longer. Polish, lacquer, and enamel are basically different words for the same product. Look for polishes with nail strengtheners and beneficial ingredients – aloe, keratin and protein. New ingredients have been developed to add strength, durability, and shine. High-priced polishes are not necessarily better than low-priced ones. Many polishes contain formaldehyde which yellows and drys nails. Its vapors may irritate the mucous membranes of the eyes, nose or mouth. Polishes are on the market that do not contain formaldehyde. If warm temperatures thicken your nail colors, keep them in a small caddy in the refrigerator.

One hundred-percent cotton balls and cotton pads absorb quickly, easily remove polish, and do not leave residual fibers. Skimpy, synthetic puffs may not as absorbent.

## The Easy Home Manicure

1. *Cuticles.* Scrub the nails with a soft brush. Soak in sudsy water to soften cuticles. Cuticle care is essential to strong nails. Massage the cuticle area. Gently push back the cuticle around the moon with an orange stick or rubber-tipped cuticle pusher. You can do this while relaxing in the bathtub. Trim only when absolutely necessary because damaging cuticles can injure the growing nail plate and lead to infection. Nip away the rough dry skin on the sides.

Apply a nail and/or cuticle conditioner. If your nails are particularly dry, reapply. Applying a conditioner on the cuticle area is beneficial even when nails are polished.

2. *Filing.* Let nails dry completely before filing or they may split. Use an emery board and file gently. Avoid filing deeply on sides. Rounded tips are easier to maintain and encourage better growth than pointed tips. To have the best shape, file them to correspond with the outline of your cuticles. Keep all nails the same length and shape. (See Illustration 27.)

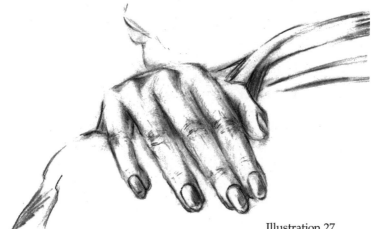

Illustration 27
Keep nails the same
length and shape

3. *Buffing.* Buff lightly from the cuticles to the tips, smoothing edges. You're buffing too hard if you feel a burning sensation. Too much buffing wears down the surface of the nails.

4. *Base Coat.* Nails must be free of any trace of polish remover. They must be clean, dry and oil-free for good adherence. Brush on a ridge-filling base if you have bumpy nails, or a nail-hardening base coat to fortify soft or weak nails. A base prevents staining, allows uniform application of nail color and "anchors" the polish so that it lasts longer.

5. *Polish.* Shaking the bottle makes bubbles which will end up on your nails. Roll it briskly between palms to thin out thickened polish. Rest your hand on a table for stability. Let the first coat dry. If the second coat is applied too soon, bubbles will occur. The second coat give the color depth and evenness and the polish lasts longer.

6. *Top Coat.* Apply a top coat or sealer. For more durability stroke it under the tips. To prevent chipping, top-coat tips frequently.

7. *Drying.* It usually takes about four hours for polish to dry hard. To expedite, you can choose one of these methods: Use a fast drying top coat or nail polish, dip nails in ice cold water for about 30 seconds, or spray with a commercial product specifically for quick drying.

A manicure is a relaxing routine, easily done while watching television, listening to the radio or reading a book. The resulting beauty confidence is well worth it. Repair chipping by touching up with polish and top coating. After a week or so, let the nails go bare a few days.

## *How to Choose the Right Colors*

Choose nail colors according to your preference, wardrobe colors and skin tone. Light complexions should avoid burgundies, maroons and browns. Most women can wear a true red. Nail color does not have to match your lips, but the shades should harmonize. Neutrals, light beiges, roses, pinks, corals, and classic reds are versatile enough to go with everything. The paler shades don't show chipping. Colors look darker in the bottle.

If your hands are (or have)…    Use…

Ruddy                           Clear red, pink-based coral, soft pink and rose. No oranges.

| | |
|---|---|
| Milky white, translucent | Soft pastels, mauve, plum, neutrals or the French manicure (tips only in beige-white, covered with a clear glaze). |
| Olive-toned | Blue-reds such as raspberry, cherry and burgundy. |
| Brown or black | Vivid shades, rich berries, wine, fuchsia, burgundy. |
| Tanned | Hot pinks, corals, orange-reds, frosts. |
| Small | Bright colors. |
| Bony | Muted colors. |
| Large | Dark shades |
| Visible veins | Avoid blue-reds; they make veins more noticeable. |
| Sallow or faded tan | Vivid shades. |
| Short, thick fingers | Flesh tones, neutrals. |
| Wide nails | Two shades same family; apply darker shade to outsides and lighter shade to middle; or don't put color all the way to the sides. |

For sheer subtlety, look for the transparencies and opalescents, or frosted translucent shades with a whisper of color.

Patricia Bozic in *30 Days to Beautiful Nails* said,"Perhaps you consider your nails details and don't want to take the time to give them the care they need....Well-groomed nails make you feel prettier and more feminine....No matter what condition yours are in right now red, ragged, ridged, split, cracked, or bitten to the quick you can make them stronger and more beautiful by following a regular nail care regime."[4]

# 9

# Accessories

Accessories extend your wardrobe by creating
the illusion of many different outfits.
Besides this, they quicken interest, spice up style,
and hint at your individual uniqueness.

Set off your fashion statement with an accessory that adds a note of fun, charm or elegance. It could be jewelry, scarves, belts, shoes, hosiery or hats.

For an outfit in shades of the same color family, accessories can be in the same family or in complementing or contrasting shades. For example, with a pink outfit wear contrasting black patent leather belt and pumps. Or, combine a bold color with a neutral. With a white jacket and cobalt blue skirt, wear a white purse and cobalt blue shoes or vice versa. Accessories pick up the colors in the outfit.

Choose accessories to play up your best features – earrings that bring out the sparkle in your eyes, elaborate rings for attractive hands, pumps to flatter shapely legs. All accessories should work with the contours of your body. If your throat is short or fleshy, wear necklines, scarves and jewelry at least four inches below the top of the collarbone to avoid a "choked-up" look. The longer throat can wear beaded, velvet choker bands, or, scarves circling the throat with a pin or clip attached.

## *Jewelry*

Large jewelry goes well with large features, but overpowers the smaller, more delicate face. One or two distinctive pieces are more elegant for special occasions than several. For the casual look and occasion, wear a variety. Flashy costume pieces like twisted metallic ropes, glass jewels in a rainbow of precious or faux stones, or spiral bracelets make old clothing look new.

Whether you should wear silver or gold depends upon skin tone and clothing colors. Some women can wear both silver and gold. Gold corresponds to the warm tones, silver to the cool ones. Go for the fun of wearing a shiny chain with casual and sporty outfits.

Luminous pearls sound a charming note for day and evening wear. They are so versatile. Wear them in twos or threes or combined with beads or scarves. Rhinestone and faceted crystal necklaces brighten evening apparel. As your budget allows, give yourself the enduring pleasure of getting a couple pieces of fine, quality jewelry.

For centuries women have worn decorations in pierced ears. The threat of losing valuable earrings is reduced, and you can still wear clipons. Medium-to-large sized button earrings with the post in the center cover wrinkled lobes. Think twice about the heavy, hanging variety that pull down the ear holes. Long earrings draw attention to the lower part of the face and the throat.

Who said earrings have to be identical? It might be better with asymmetrical hairstyles to have a bigger adornment on one ear than on the other. With multiple colors in dressing you may want earrings to pick up several colors.

Pins express your mood and individuality. Use them on hip pockets, belts or in clusters. Place a dramatic or heirloom piece near or on the shoulder to top a suit.

## Eyeglasses

For most women, glasses are our most important accessory. Actually, they are necessary accessories. They make work and play one hundred percent easier. The right frames with the right lenses can add distinction and character to all faces.

We talk to the eyes and subtle color makes them more attractive. Lenses tend to obscure the eyes. Add clarity by lining the upper and lower lids and lighten the eye area with a pale shadow and a generous application of mascara. If eye makeup is not an option, wear lipstick and blush.

If you are farsighted, the lenses of your glasses make eyes look larger. If you are nearsighted, the lenses make eyes look smaller.

*Frames.* Because people often see the glasses before the eyes, shop for the best fitting frames that complement all your features and hair. Insist that they don't slip down but rest on the nose not on the cheeks. The pupils of the eyes should appear in the center of the lenses or near to it.

Upward-tilting frames or high temples provide a lift at the sides of the face. The upper parts should follow the natural line of the brows. For crow's-feet, opt for side pieces hooked to the top and bottom of the lenses. A low bridge breaks the vertical line of a long nose. Sometimes rimless frames make the face look older.

### Guidelines for Selecting Frames

| If your face is: | Frames should be: |
| --- | --- |
| Oval | Squarish, usually any style but extremes. Rimless is good. With a very thin oval face, use frames for the oblong/rectangle shape. |
| Square | Soft or rounded edges. |
| Rectangular | Angular to shorten a long face and wide at checkbones. Decorative sidebars. |

Round                    Angular or hexagonal, not round.
Inverted Triangle        Round or square.
Fair Complexion          Lightweight metals or plastic in crystal or
                         light shades
Dark Complexion          Bright metallics like white gold, pink
                         lilac, raspberry, emerald.

*Sunglasses.* According to the American Academy of Ophthalmology,[1] studies reveal that large amounts of visible blue, violet and invisible ultraviolet light that are found in sunlight can be harmful to the eyes. They accelerate the aging and deterioration of human vision and play a major role in the formation of cataracts.

To avoid color distortion and still have good screening from ultraviolet A and B (UVA and UVB) rays, lenses in dark grey, green or a combination with brown have proven to be satisfactory. Lenses tinted pink, purple, and especially blue distort color perception (for example traffic lights) and are not usually dark enough for effective blocking. Look for the words "special

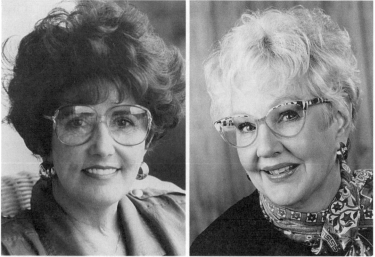

Frames courtesy of              Frames courtesy of
Optical Sales, Portland, OR     Europtics, Inc. Denver, CO

Your face deserves a flattering frame.

purpose" or "blocks 99 percent of ultraviolet (UV) rays." Some block 100 percent. "Cosmetic" or "fashion" sunglasses block 70 percent or less.

Wraparound sunglasses prevent ultraviolet light from sneaking past the top, bottom and sides. The best are snug-fitting or curved to fit the face, with opaque or ultraviolet blocking side shields.

## Scarves

For decades, scarves have been the trademarks of Sparky, a writer and teacher who lives in the farm country of Washington State. She has several dozen rectangular, circular and square scarves from many countries. With dresses, skirts and blouses she wears exotic ones. For work she has color coded them for each task – yellow for mowing grass, blue for hen-house clean-ing, lavender for tidying the barn, red for picking berries, cerise for weeding (she hates weeding and loves cerise), orange for sweeping the walks and porches, flamboyant pink for washing windows, and brown for working with the bees.

She wrote in a newspaper article about one morning when she was wearing an old gray sweatshirt over pedal pushers, a varicolored green scarf covering curlers, and a matching scarf around her throat. It was tied in back, the ends fluttering in the breeze as she pushed a wheelbarrow of horse droppings to fertilize the flower garden. Her neighbor, a retired doctor and not a well man, smiled as he watched and leaned over the fence. "Sparky, it's amazing how charming you look when you're hauling manure. You always make me feel better when I see you in one of your beautiful scarves."

With her mania for scarves, her husband thinks that some-how Sparky, now 80, always looks prettier than other women.[2]

Select these fun-filled accessories to pick up the colors of your clothing or to add a note of contrast. To be a true comple-ment to your costume, they must look like an integral part, not like an afterthought.

Chiffon, silk, and lightweight polyesters in brights, pastels, neutrals or woven with sparkling threads are kind to the face. Equally eyecatching are scarves in paisleys, geometrics, florals or plaids. Printed scarves go with prints in clothing if the shades are identical. For example, a scarf or tie splashed with red and white polka dots adds a jaunty touch to a red and white striped blouse or dress.

> If your scarf tends to wander from
> its best position, anchor it under your
> garment with a safety pin.

Try this graceful frame for the face. Fold a large square silk or chiffon scarf into a triangle, and place it around your throat. Pull the two ends of the long edge through a scarf clip. Place the "V" in back and adjust the loose ends under the chin or drape them over a shoulder. Wear over a sweater or dress, or with a jacket. You can also add glitter by wearing a necklace that picks up the colors of the scarf, chain(s) or pearls.

Even more interesting is a combination of different fabric textures, such as a silk chiffon scarf woven with a metallic thread over a casual knit, or a frothy lace scarf with a denim jacket, shirt and/or jeans.

For the sophisticated, cavalier look, fold a silk scarf like a cravat inside an open-necked cotton shirt or jacket. (See Illustration 28.)

*More Scarf Tips.* Enfold your favorite long chain in a scarf as you drape it around your throat. To cover a wrinkled throat, wrap a small rectangular scarf around twice and tie in front or on the side. Option: Fasten with your favorite clip or pin.

When using a scarf for contrast or as an accent, let your lip color and nail polish pick up the accent color.

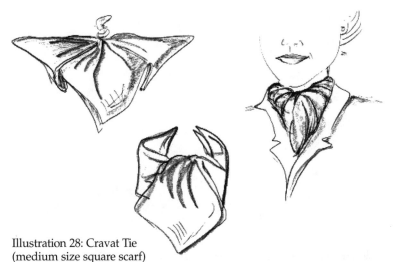

Illustration 28: Cravat Tie
(medium size square scarf)
Gather up four or five inches of the center; tie in a knot; spread out like a diamond with the knot underneath; pick up two opposite corners and place around your throat, tie in back, tuck in knot.

If you have a jacket with a low neckline, use it to showcase a flashy oblong scarf and/or an heirloom pendant. (See Illustrations 29, 30, 31.)

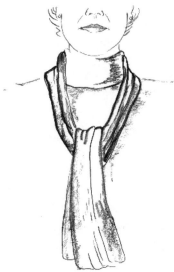

Illustration 29: Oblong Flip
(36" or larger oblong scarf)
For added flair, embellish with a chain, pearls or beads.

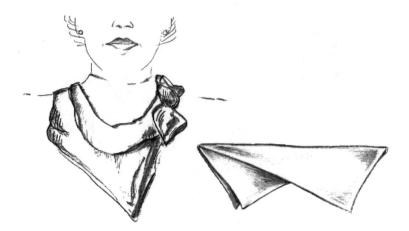

Illustration 30: Versatile Collar (36" or larger square scarf)
Fold square in half to form a rectangle. Then fold diagonally to form
one straight edge and two points. Drape straight edge around shoulders.
Bring two ends of the straight edge together at front and tie in a square
knot—right over left then left over right. Wear with knot in front, on
shoulder or in the back.

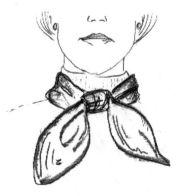

Illustration 31: Oblong Tie (short or long oblong scarf)
Tie a loose half knot at the place where you want the knot to appear
at the center of the throat. Bring the other end around the neck and pull it
through the loop of the knot. Adjust tightness.

## Ties

What an exciting accessory! Remember those old pictures of schoolmarms with straight black ties, white shirts and long black skirts? Today a revolution has changed ties for women. The fabric is a lovely silk in unbelievably beautiful colors. It's fun to wear a flashy tie to brighten up a somber suit. It can express the fun, glamour or conservative aspect of your personality. Contrasts are wonderful!

## Hats

Like scarves, wear hats to match your outfit in style, color and mood. The shape of a hat should complement the contours of your face. Please note the photograph on page 175.

## Handbags

They don't have to match your shoes. The most popular choice is one with lots of utilitarian pockets in a taupe, saddle brown, black or any neutral that goes with everything. The size of the handbag should be in proportion to the size of the figure. Many women opt for large bags regardless. For special occasions, the shallow, small purse goes well with the petite figure and a larger bag for the woman who is over five-foot-five. The more formal the occasion, the simpler the bag.

*Totes.* Tote-toting women are happy women. They have everything their life depends upon in that wonderful tote – well, almost everything. Totes have become *the* essential accessory. They offer an explosion of exciting patterns and compositions – plain canvas with bright trim, bold graphics, a pageant of floral blossoms against pastels or white, giant daisies on brown, the posh one-color leather or exotic skins. Many women are acquiring a wardrobe of totes to house their necessities and to go out and about with that wonderful feeling, "I have everything I need."

## *Hosiery*

The choices have increased with every decade. Besides pantyhose, we have leggings (no feet in them), tights, trouser socks, sport socks, and knee-highs. Styles for socks include crew, fitness, hiking, athletic and walking. And a wide array of textures and prints are available, such as flowered, Mickey Mouse, lace jersey, embroidered, rib knit, silk blends, cotton cable, and Lycra.

Tights come in silken crochet, openwork, fishnet, faux fishnet, or textures in honeycomb, daisy and diamond. With skorts, shorts, and short skirts, wear leggings with socks, tights, or pantyhose for slicker-looking legs. Both tights and pantyhose have control tops to smooth out the tummy and hide the panty line under slacks. Match them to your outfit or select neutrals. Black leggings look good on all body types except skinny. When they fit well, they last. For pumping iron and exercise walking, nothing beats the comfort of a sweat shirt, shorts, leggings, roll-up socks and sport shoes.

I met a snazzy 70-plus athlete who race-walked in the Senior Games. She wore a black hip-high body suit with suntan tights. When a friend admired her sylphlike figure, she said with a twinkle in her eyes, "I love tights. They sure do firm up the flab!" How true! How true!

What a variety there is to give us good-looking legs! Deep-hued hosiery thins legs. Some brands have pantyhose for full figures that need extra stretch in the waist, hips and thighs. These styles give all-day comfort and a good fit. Light shades give body to thin legs. The one-tonal look from leg to foot is a figure-flattering, pulled-together style. Match hem and hose, or hose and shoes. Either way, it is a classy touch.

## *Suggestions for Matching Hose and Shoes*

| Shoes | Hose |
|---|---|
| Sport shoes | Socks, leggings with socks |
| Slip-ons or flats | Opaque or sheer, tights, knee-hi's |

| | |
|---|---|
| Oxfords | Tights, pantyhose, knee-highs, bright or dark shades or same color as shoes, opaque |
| Pumps | Opaque or sheer |
| Dressy sandals | Sheer |
| Boots | Tights or hose to match hem or boots |

## *Shoes*

Shoes are smart updaters. Top priorities are comfort and a good fit. Sport shoes of all types, such as Reboks, Nikes and tennis shoes, are favorites for more than sports and exercising. It has become the in-thing to wear them for shopping, conventions, or rushing from office to office. Women in smartly-styled suits and dresses with designer purses are choosing sport shoes for their walking trips. What a wonderful commonsense switch in fashion!

When you shop for shoes and want a true fit, it helps to remember that feet swell as the day goes on. If possible, do it before midafternoon. Soft leather uppers mold to the irregularities of the foot. Leather soles conform better than non-leather. They are lightweight, bend easier and, if stitched, show top quality.

Ever-smart spectator pumps are worn year-round in combinations, such as taupe with black, black with brown, red with black, bluette with black, or cream or white with black. Stylish shoes now have comfortable heels. Silver and gold flats, luxurious loafers in reptilian skins, and suede or patent in multiple colors spruce up any outfit. Shoes in reds, emeralds, purples, turquoise or pastels give zing to your fashion statement and put spring in your step.

# 10

# Restoring a Positive Image After Mastectomy and Ileostomy

> "I believe that it is possible to find
> some joy in almost every experience....
> What is a happy ending? Is it having
> a face without wrinkles? Is it never
> being ill or disappointed? Is it never los-
> ing a loved one? I think not. For me, a
> happy ending is the knowledge that,
> even though the flame may flicker, my
> inner candle of joy burns brightly."
> —Lois Tschetter Hjelmstad
> *Fine Black Lines*
> *Reflections on Facing Cancer, Fear and Loneliness*[1]

Although this chapter refers to mastectomy and ostomy, I hope all women facing any kind of defeminizing surgery and their friends and relatives will be helped by its ideas. My research reveals that practically everyone knows someone who has had or will have this experience.

## *Mastectomy*

When I met the author of the above quotation, her first words after the usual pleasantries were, "Why don't you write something for women like me?" Her book, *Fine Black Lines*, chronicles her life with cancer through journal entries, essays and poetry. Ever since she was a girl, she has used poetry to think through the gamut of her emotions. Cancer intensified that process, leaving her with a strong desire to help smooth the road for women like her.

I interviewed women from her cancer support group to find out how they kept "the candle of joy" burning after the devastation of losing one or both breasts. The solution, they said, is to work constantly at having useful lives and to stay on the lighter side as much as possible. These women found that being part of a support group was indispensable. The comraderie helped tremendously. They hunt for humor, squeeze joy and rewards from every day, and get together to laugh about a gorgeous prosthesis or cry over a discouraging prognosis. Sharing the good and the bad, they feel like extended family, bonded by common experience and caring understanding.

The women I met were attractive and working in the mainstream. Although they grieve silently for their loss, they keep busy recreating meaningful lives. Many things were important during their healing processes. Here are some of them:

- *Set priorities.* Knowing their energy would be low, they set priorities. Life had to be simpler, uncomplicated. They had to decide what they had to do and what someone else could do for them. Someone else could clean their houses, prepare food, shop for groceries, handle bills and insurance. Personal appearance was up to them.

- *Will.* They found the strength to push themselves to do the things they had to do. One was addressing an audience when a hot flash overwhelmed her. She felt perspiration beads on her face as the heat rushed through it. Forcing herself to control every aspect of her presentation, she succeeded without a glitch. She found out that when she doubted she could do some task, she could make herself stop doubting and just do it. Anticipating the healing power of active living and a good attitude, these women will themselves to be pleasant when they do not feel like it and to do when they don't think they can.

- *Appearance.* Another woman said she didn't want people thinking, "That poor thing!" She wanted to look healthy. Looking her best reinforced her. "I feel less vulnerable to the world," she said. It empowered her when she was dealing with people in her business and it was one less worry. Presenting a positive image captured a firmer sense of normalcy. Many of these women found that even when they could hardly raise a brush to their hair, the effort to look their best made for a happier day.

- *Smile!* Smiling empowers. One woman said it made her happy when people smiled back and were pleasant to her. She felt like she was a mirror and people reflected her smile and good humor.

- *No one can read your mind!* Tell your friends, associates and relatives exactly what you need. They want direction to help, even if it is just conversation – non-personal talk, talking about anything but *the* problem. If you want relief from talking or thinking about it, tell them.

- *Faith.* Seek all the spiritual and material help that is available. Be patient and loving with yourself and everyone. Your good friends and relatives will enjoy the feeling of being needed and able to help.

They all agreed that when life is threatened it becomes more precious. The urge is to live it fully. A good appearance and planned activity, working or volunteering, are crucial to mind/body healing. Working outside the home during chemotherapy and recovery was literally lifesaving to many of them. Helping and being with people was like a warm spring breeze on a cold winter day.

Conclusion. Striving to heal mind and body, striving to keep the candle of joy burning brightly, brings us out of the fog of despair into the sunshine of victory.

### Reconstructive Surgery

Recent developments and new procedures have evolved remarkable physical and psychological transformation through reconstructive breast surgery. The skill and experience of the surgeon cannot be overemphasized. Breast reconstruction is a very emotional decision. A woman needs a doctor who takes time to be attentive to her concerns and treats her as an individual.

Dr. Douglas McKinnon is a plastic and reconstructive surgeon, certified by the American Society of Plastic and Reconstructive Surgeons, Inc. Modern breast reconstruction goes back 15 years and Doctor McKinnon has been involved since then. The choice for reconstruction after mastectomy is highly personal. Some women do well without it and do not wish to subject themselves to more surgery. Others want to look in the mirror and see their body as natural as possible. There are different reliable procedures that meet their psychological and aesthetic expectations.

More often than not the operation is done in multiple stages and does not have to be complex or require lots of time off for recuperation. Reconstructions are different in feel and texture but even with minimal clothing they can look quite normal. Many women have had breast reconstruction and feel their body is whole again without the constant reminder of mastectomy.

Dr. McKinnon recommends *A Woman's Decision Breast Care, Treatment, and Reconstruction* by Karen Berger, a nurse, and John Bostwick III, M.D. It is enlightening even if reconstruction is not a consideration. The text is thorough, excellent, and easy-to-read. Explanations present commonsense answers to the apprehensions of women and to the questions of men who love their women and want to know how to intelligently help with decisions, how to play the role of supporting player, how to deal with sex and many other anxieties.

### The Lingerie Solution

Every woman can find beautiful lingerie to fit her physical and emotional requirements. Understanding attendants in special shops, often found in or near hospitals, help sensitive and reluctant women who need guidance. Different styles offer choices that will give you comfort and self-assurance.

Women with single mastectomies can use their own brassieres or any bra and place a prosthesis in the cup. They can also purchase a brassiere with a pocket for the prosthesis. Pocket brassieres come in many colors, styles and fabrics, even pretty laces. They are also worn by women who have had bilateral mastectomies.

The self-attachment prosthesis system contains adhesive supports that affix to the skin; Velcro on the other side holds the prostheses. It can be worn with or without a bra and under swimsuits and strapless gowns.

Another choice is the cotton polyester camisole with satin ribbon detailing and interior pockets that hold breast forms in various sizes and shapes. Smoothly and gently covering the surgical area, it can be worn from hospital to home. These shops stock complete lines of mastectomy products including swimwear, wigs, turbans, and nightgowns. Silk underwear, T-shirts and pajamas are soothing on the skin and give a feeling of gentleness and being pampered. You need that now!

### Hair

Products that promote healthy hair and scalp, especially for women who are going through chemotherapy, are available in upscale salons. With some combinations of chemo drugs, hair loss is certain. When you are advised that it is, get a wig before the process begins. Match it exactly to your hair or get an exciting change...blond or red? Choose one that complements your skin. If you wish, have it styled by a hairdresser.

Some chapters of the American Cancer Society have wig banks that supply them at no charge. For additional information call 1-800-ACS-2345 or your local ACS chapter. Some specialty shops have wig kits that have shampoo, conditioner and instructions on how to take care of them. When the scalp gets hot or sensitive from wearing one, freshen and remove excess oil with a mild shampoo.

*Turbans, Scarves and Caps.* Caps, either designer or sporty, appear more normal than turbans or scarves. Turbans and caps are more user-friendly because it is difficult to raise the arms after surgery. Go for cheerful, becoming colors and you can accessorize with pins and matching earrings.

### Cosmetic Tattooing

Cosmetic tattooing gives permanent eye lining and brows and helps to relieve anxiety when hair loss is certain. Results can be very satisfying but proceed with caution. Consult *only* with a *cosmetic* tattooist who is recommended by a board certified plastic surgeon or your State Board of Cosmetology. The process is safe when done by a qualified cosmetic tattooist. She should be attentive to your desires and use the color that will always be attractive. This will conserve energy and it give you the comfort of knowing your face has brows and your eyes are defined until hair grows back. Look into this before chemotherapy when nerves are more stable. See chapter 3 for more information.

### Skin Care

Whatever your skin was, it will be dry and sensitive after chemotherapy. Even oily skin becomes dry. Exfoliators and masks improve the texture. Using one of these products removes surface sludge, enabling a moisturizer to be more effectively absorbed and gives your complexion a healthy glow. Deodorants, shaving, saunas, Jacuzzis, loofahs, strong soaps, even washcloths can be problematical.

*Cleansing.* Use a gentle liquid face and body cleanser, formulated for dry skin. No hot water. Take slightly warm showers and baths. A cool bath with a bit of safflower or sunflower oil is refreshing.

*Moisturizing.* Avoid heavy oils. Keep skin moist with lightweight moisturizers such as these dermatologist recommended moisturizers: Cetaphil, Moisturel, Candermyl, Replenaderm, and Eucerin. One that is too heavy may cause breakouts and cremes are oilier than lotions. Use plant oils – olive, safflower, sunflower – for dry patches. If it has a sun protection factor, that is even better. Keep all products out of the eyes.

*Sunscreen.* Chemotherapeutic agents usually cause photosensitivity and an impaired immune system. Exposure to harmful UVA and UVB rays of the sun makes the skin vulnerable. A sunscreen, without strong chemicals like PABA, protects and prevents discolorations from getting darker. The inert chemical, microfine titanium dioxide, is the active ingredient that blocks out UVA, UVB and visible light. You can also get sun protection in moisturizers, lip balms, lipsticks and foundations.

## Makeup

To avoid infection, discard old makeup and start anew. Use cotton balls and disposable applicators. If you use brushes, cleanse weekly and soak in alcohol. Never share makeup, a good rule for all of us. The focal point of your appearance is the face, not the torso. Makeup beautifies. With minimal effort you will get maximum benefit. Wear only your best warm (yellow based) or cool (pink/blue based) colors. When you see the glowing result of subtle color, correctly blended, it boosts morale.

*Concealants.* Cancer treatments may change skin to sallow, ruddy or pale and/or cause hyper-pigmentation (dark spots). Quality concealants and foundations hide imperfections. Apply a concealant on spots, add a whisper of powder for staying power, then foundation over the entire face.

*Foundation.* A quality foundation or base that gives good coverage is an additional protection from the sun and adds a flawless even tone. Too light a shade looks chalky or ashy. Select a shade that enriches.

*Defining the Eyes.* Brow and lashes grow back fast. In the meantime, you can enhance your eyes with these tips. The dark line created by lashes, not their length, defines the eyes. The glue used for false lashes may be irritating, especially if eyes feel dry and sensitive. Eye lining, like all facial colorings, should harmonize with the skin and other makeup and not grab attention. Remember the raccoon! Black eye lining with ice blue eyes is overpowering and diminishes their beauty. A muted color goes better with the pale iris. Liners come in different shades sage, grey, taupe, brown and ebony. Brown is a popular choice. Line lower lids along the roots of the lashes, and the uppers if it is easy for you, to within one-half to one-quarter of an inch from the inner corners. In case hot flashes brought on by menopausal symptoms washes away eye lining, try using an eyelining pen, rather than pencil, or waterproof mascara, applying it with a small brush.

*Brows.* They are easily added or thickened by using either a brow pencil or powder. Brow powders and gels from Borghese, Ultima II, and Lancôme give a softer look. For the natural brow line, define three points on the brow bone: the inner one over the inner eye corner, the midpoint over the pupil of the eye as you look straight into the mirror and the outer point. To find the outer point, take a pencil and hold it from the edge of the nose to the outer corner of the eyes. The place where it touches the brow bone is the outer point. Connect these points by stroking in color, building it to natural-looking thickness. Check an old photo for the best shape.

*Shadow.* Use matte, fragrance-free and non-drying eye shadows. Shadow is shading, which means keep it muted. Taupe, buff, peach, bamboo, ivory, sand, pink, gray, mushroom, ginger and brown are good colors if they flatter hair, skin and eyes darker – skin tones take darker colors.

*Cheeks.* Do not use browns or neutrals. Select rose, mauve, terra-cotta, peach, coral or whatever color brightens the eyes and harmonizes with your skin tones. Blend carefully so it is not a blob but a natural looking glow on your cheeks. Let it look like it comes from the inside out. This calls for subtle, flattering color and diminishing the hue into the foundation.

*Lips.* Lips may be very dry. Apply either a lip balm with sunscreen or Vaseline. Let absorb. Then, line lips to get the shape you want and fill in with an emollient lipstick. *The less lipstick you apply to get the best color, the longer it will stay on.* A lip brush controls the amount of color and easily blends it into the outline.

### Nails

For dry, brittle nails, use a cuticle conditioner/moisturizer to alleviate dehydration. If your oncologist approves, massage the cuticle area with an 8 percent alpha hydroxy acid moisturizing creme. Do not use nail wraps. Keep nails shaped and avoid buffing which thins. Never cut or severely push back cuticles because of possible infection.

### Scent Sense

According to an ancient proverb, Every perfume is a medicine. The perfumes, colognes and essences of today have progressed from being just pretty fragrances to their age-old mission of evoking relaxation, rejuvenation, well-being, even clarity of thought. As subtly as the breath of spring flowers, the scents we love quietly imitate part of our Self.

## *Ileostomy*

Carol had ulcerative colitis. There was no known cause. The only treatment was total removal of the large intestine, which required an exterior opening in the abdomen and forces her to wear an appliance. It changed her whole body image.

The years after the operation were very difficult. She was a closet ostomate (one who has an artificial passage for elimination). She felt like a freak, not wanting to talk about it to anyone including her family. It was like a horse on a coffee table – everyone knows it's there, but no one wants to say it is.

"That was sick," Carol said. "A feeling of privacy is one thing, but wanting to hide it or thinking I'm a freak is sick." She thought her children's friends would make fun of her. So, they pretended there were no problems.

Along with self-depreciation and the family's reluctance to discuss anything negative, she tried to cope with an alcoholic husband whom she loved, depression, smoking, Valium, self-medication – the whole unhappy cycle. She did not know how to be open about her struggle. The closed-family thinking kept her husband and children from talking about their worries and sharing honest feelings.

"I could have helped them with their fears and they could have given me some strokes that I needed so badly. I did not know how to allow their goodness to come to me," she said. No doctor ever suggested counseling. She thought it was crazy to go to a therapist.

After 19 years, at 48, Carol was shocked into reality when she screamed her rage and helplessness at her husband. She committed herself for 30 days to a drug/alcohol treatment center. She said it was a spiritual quest as much as anything and she received the awakening she sought. "Getting this treatment was the biggest and best turning point in my life," she said. "I gave up Valium cold turkey and smoking one year later."

Although it is still difficult for her to refer to her surgery and appliance, she no longer feels like a freak. She is divorced, but happier about herself than at any other time in her life. Both children are back living with her. They can talk about the bad stuff and the ever-growing good stuff. There are no longer any bad habits and if that horse ever shows up on the coffee table again, they are ready to talk about it. They do not have to pretend.

Carol feels that some kind of counseling to build self-appreciation is very important after surgical trauma, especially if the patient has low self-esteem to begin with. As for her appearance, the appliance does not show; there are no bulges. She wears a light panty girdle or control top pantyhose (after checking with her doctor to be sure the pressure was okay). Both are comfortable. She wears anything but a bikini – even straight skirts and flat front jeans.

"We don't have to wear shapeless clothes like blouses hanging outside skirts or slacks. I find that looking my best is vitally important to my emotional health. We need that during and after recovery, and we need to fight depression. Looking as attractive as we can is one way to do it."

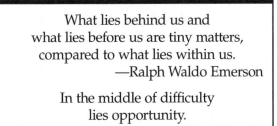

What lies behind us and
what lies before us are tiny matters,
compared to what lies within us.
—Ralph Waldo Emerson

In the middle of difficulty
lies opportunity.
—Albert Einstein

## Relax? How?

Walking, exercising, physical activities are part of the solution, and deep breathing is another, soothing body and mind. Try this: Inhale with a slight outward push in the abdomen, take the breath up expanding the rib cage, filling the lungs and exhale slowly. Do it several times a day, especially when fears pester you. Notice how deep breathing corrects posture, too.

Women have found in meditation a new peaceful state that helps them to think clearly, lowers pressures and destresses. Bookstores and libraries have tapes on relaxation and meditation techniques.

## *Create a Life!* _____

Play a musical instrument, paint/sketch a picture, read a humorous or enthralling book, plan regular walks in the park, write in a daily journal, set new goals, volunteer, work at something, etc. Keep active. Do not isolate yourself. People are important to happiness, and you are important to them... you are.

Start writing two to three pages a day in your *private* journal for no one's eyes but yours. Stretch it to three a day even if you write an affirmation, an uplifting thought, or a happy memory five or six times. This is your confessional. Cry over it if you wish. If you love poetry, try it. How well you write doesn't matter. Only you see it. Put your thoughts, feelings, fears and hopes on paper. It is a dynamic, surprisingly subtle way to heal and regenerate yourself. Lots of people, men and women, who want to create a good life use this tool and it works.

Sue Buchanan, author of *Love, Laughter and A High Disregard for Statistics Surviving breast cancer with your sense of humor and your sexuality intact,* writes about creating a life and celebrating it. After months of aggressive chemotherapy, she happened to see her doctor's notes. They said she wouldn't live more than a year and would not be a good candidate for breast reconstruction. That was over 11 years ago! Since then, she did have a successful breast reconstruction, continues to work her career and help women. To everyone, she says, there is life – *a lot of life* – during and after cancer.

# Epilogue

## Birthdays Don't Count!

"The young are beautiful,
but the old are more
beautiful than the young."
—Walt Whitman[1]

Why shouldn't personal beauty remain part of a long life? More and more women are realizing that beauty is appropriate all our years and *we are aging younger.* This realization is regenerating. It lifts our spirits to know we can add life to our appearance and feel good about it. This recreation of ourselves has no relevance to a birth date. So, why not develop a master plan of individual style that reflects an ageless attitude?

Suppose you are discouraged or just bored with the way you look, where do you begin? Start by tossing out the old stuff. Go through closets and drawers and give away everything that even hints of the matronly, dowdy or outmoded. If you haven't worn something for two to three years, trash it. It's just taking up space. The same goes for cosmetics. Get rid of those you haven't worn. They do nothing for you, and that's why you instinctively don't wear them. Make room for makeup that enhances your natural beauty, and fashions with flair as well as comfort.

Spend quiet time thinking about the new you. Release your imagination and listen to your intuitive, artistic sense. If you are in earnest, ideas will start percolating. Experiment with new techniques, new products, new colors. Feel the energy of getting out of that "old" rut! If we ever needed newness, it is now.

When we remove limitations, we have no idea what doors will open, what dreams will be realized. We "lose ourselves" in grandchildren, painting, music, gardening, career, romance, etc., but we find ourselves when we discover our individual specialness and the beauty potential that's been hiding behind old habits. A new career or enterprise, a new talent or hobby, enjoyable new friends, an exciting adventure, or unexpected opportunity are waiting for you when you are receptive to them. Your new mode will facilitate the happening. This is not "pie in the sky," but you won't know for sure unless you try it, will you?

The way you dress expresses not only your personality but how you feel about yourself, and frequently, how you feel about other people. Personal style is influenced by your sense of what's appropriate and best for your individuality, comfort zone, style of living, and the occasion.

When you decide to put pizazz into your appearance, give serious thought to the following concepts:

**Don't dress according to your age.** How often we get caught into that common mind trap, "I would love to wear that, but I'm just too old." Nonsense! Being over 50, 60, 70, or whatever the number doesn't mean we have to dress older. Of course, there are certain things we may not want to wear, such as showing too much bare skin, wearing midthigh skirts, or figure-revealing styles. But, that leaves lots of room for elegance, glamour and fun-to-wear apparel. Our distinctive style and color personality still needs to be expressed. Forget the number. Instead, let what you wear say who you are, not how old.

In a wardrobe planning class a woman who was 26 said she was serious about her career, but was unhappy because people thought she was 18 and treated her as though she was. She wanted to look older. We encouraged her to dress, not "older," but more conservatively and develop a sophistication that communicates maturity.

By contrast, consider my friend, Orra, who was pushing 70 but looking fiftyish. She appeared ageless. Petite with reddish-brown hair, she expressed an abundance of charisma, grace and disciplined professionalism. With her faultless application of makeup, simple but smart fashions, erect posture and congeniality, she was a true gentlewoman. For many years she owned and operated her own real estate agency and was the first woman to be elected president of the state board of realtors when she was almost 70. "Always look 10 to 20 years younger than you are," she counseled. She knew that appearance was a decisive factor in setting our stage for success...success in every avenue of life and especially in a competitive environment.

Look at Barbara Walters, Debbie Reynolds, Candice Bergen, and Cher – all are over 50. Celebrities do us a tremendous favor. They exemplify the new concept of enduring vitality that far surpasses the old thought of passivity. Their positive, distinctive style shows us the way to go.

Donna Karan, fashion designer with The Donna Karan Company, New York City, said, "I don't think it [fashion and image] has anything to do with your age; I think it has to do with your state of mind. I see women in their fifties and sixties who are totally ageless...and look snazzy and...marvelous."[2]

**Figure problems are not reasons to be unattractive.** Beauty comes in all sizes and shapes. Fat or thin, short or tall does not determine our beauty potential, but self-thought does. Never forfeit the development of your stunning style to imperfections of the body. Accept the challenge to look your best and you will when you really want it.

The fashion industry designs for size 16 and over. By using compatible colors and couturier lines, as described in Chapter 8, we give balance to our profile. Dresses with large bold colorful prints give a striking look to the oversized woman, as do slimming one-color suits.

**Be dramatic with fashion when the occasion or your desire calls for it.** Try striking combinations of color, such as turquoise with fuchsia, fuchsia or red with yellow, coral with turquoise, or forest green with bright purple. The color plates in fashion magazines illustrate energizing color mixes.

**If your legs are slender and pretty, wear the higher hems.** For the petite figure, leg-lengthening two-inch high heels are becoming and feminine. She should also keep the hem mid-knee especially if her legs are short. Otherwise, her figure looks dumpy. Go for elegant, delicate, provocative and trend-setting fabrics and styles if they are your forté and fit your comfort zone. Try the fun and flair of mixing the elegant with the casual – a lace or chiffon shirt with blue jeans; a filmy chiffon shirt with a tailored or pleated skirt; a ribbed cashmere sweater over a brocade skirt. Experience the versatile Chanel jacket over shorts, long dresses, flippy skirts and even jeans. It's okay to break free of confining concepts to wear sequins to the casual or sporty event, and sweaters for galas, if that suits your fancy. Listen to your intuition, and create pleasure-giving clothing combinations.

**Liberate your personal sense of beauty.** Convince yourself that you are getting better every day, not the opposite! Put forth your best, most colorful image in either ethereal pastels, vivid brights, rich deep tones, earthy hues, or striking monochromatic combos. Open your mind to that timeless, beautiful woman inside and let her out!

**Be recreative about yourself.** What a lift this gives our spirit! Some people think appearance is superficial, but if you think about it, you will realize that appearance is a direct reflection of how you see yourself and that is how you will be seen. When you look in the mirror, ask yourself: Does this reflection represent the true me? Is this the persona I want to project?

**Once you've done your beauty work, forget the body and enjoy the flow of life.** To constantly worry if your hair is right, if your lipstick is still on, if the slip is hanging or all the other ifs only adds another wrinkle. You checked everything, right? Now, forget it. Eliminate appearance anxiety. You're all right. To become an image addict, always checking for imperfections, is as bad as never doing it. Work with your intuition, expand your self-awareness and stick like fly paper to your progress in beauty awareness.

**Be discriminating about image advice.** You are the ultimate expert. The guidelines throughout this book are just that – guidelines to help you achieve the image you want. They are not inflexible. If you bend the basics and put together a smashing statement of personal style that beckons compliments and makes you feel good, congratulate yourself. The first point is perhaps the most important: Calendar age has little to do with the attractive, timeless you.

## *How to Find Your Best Overall Look*

Your best look is a union of what's current and what's you. Nancy Taylor Farel, Boulder, Colorado, is in the business of helping women and men develop their best look. She specializes in personal colors and wardrobe consulting for individuals and corporations. Nancy has seen from experience, and corporate executives have told her, that people appreciate a woman more and react positively when her appearance expresses the vital person she is. "The rewarding experiences and compliments we get when we look our best – at any age – give us a lift that has nothing to do with ego. To get lazy about appearance is to miss this benefit," she said.

Appearance expresses the person you are and what you do. Because women in their 50s often have a different agenda, a different mode of life, from women who are over 60, we offer two different slants toward expressing your winning look. Because the lifestyle of women in their 50s and those who are 60+ can be different, Nancy suggests ideas to accommodate both groups. These may overlap for most women. For example, laser resurfacing and sunscreen are options for all women over 50. There are no carved-in-cement limits to any age group.

*For Women in Their 50s.* Fashion your appearance toward achieving your goals in life. Your job or career is a major influence on your wardrobe.

- Definitely look into retin A and alpha hydroxy acid products. They maintain a smooth complexion. You may want to investigate laser resurfacing.

- Wear foundation and makeup because the finished, polished look diminishes signs of aging. You are competing with younger women in the marketplace. For dry skin, use a moisturizer and most women find sunscreen a necessity. Makeup tones should be appropriate for your job. Save dramatic colors, especially in eye shadow, for evenings.

- In the workplace, avoid noisy jewelry, mini skirts, sleeveless tops, lace, patterned or bright colored hose. Wear a good, supporting bra and control top panty hose.

- Dress for comfort. Give the "sit test" to every skirt to be sure exposure is controlled. Tight is not sexy. It is uncomfortable and inappropriate when working. Save very feminine apparel for evenings. Your appearance is an influential sidebar to your capability on the job and to your economic advancement.

*For Women Over 60.* Define your lifestyle and keep appearance up-to-date. You need a versatile wardrobe to suit your various activities, that may include a career or part-time work, along with volunteering, community activities, sports, travel, etc.

- Use regularly retin-A and/or an AHA lotion/creme that is compatible with your skin.

- Sunscreen is necessary, especially if you like to soak in the sun. Your skin is more susceptible to burning because it has less protecting melanin. Wear a three-inch brim hat either designer or sporty.

- Check your foundation color to be sure it is not chalky or dry looking.

- Your face has more vitality if you use a slightly richer shade in blush and lipstick.

- Avoid bright shades in eye shadow. Subtle eye lining gives more definition to eyes behind glasses. Lash primers are an undercoat for fine, thin lashes. They help to build, thicken and condition. Take a look at Estee Lauder's Primer, Lancôme's Forticils or Origins' Underwear for Lashes.

- As hair color lightens, update the color of your brow pencil/powder/gel to go with it. Brows that are too light or too dark do nothing to beautify your face.

- Update your hairstyle! A hairdo with up-swing and becoming color is definitely de-aging.

*More tips for the savvy woman:*

- Investigate the gentle lightweight undergarments in lingerie departments that nip in the midriff, waist and tummy. Choices vary from moderate to firm control and from briefs to pantylegs.

- Casual does not mean sloppy.

- Body-hugging shoulder pads keeps the lines of your garments crisp.

- Tight clothing makes you look larger.

- Go for relaxed design rather than too much structure, such as a fitted suit, unless you have an elegant figure.

- For the full-figured woman, keep pins, broaches and scarves around the shoulder line not the bust.

- Eye glasses are the one accessory that is indispensable and everyone notices. Keep the frames modern. Lenses are less apparent with anti-reflective (AR) coating because it reduces glare. It also eases eye strain from computer work and night driving.

The purpose of makeup and fashion is not to create a stylized manikin. It is to highlight the beauty of the person you are.

Isn't panache a wonderful word? It is much more colorful than "flair" or "dash." What a lift to the spirit to have at least one outfit with panache! An outfit with panache perfectly mirrors and uniquely magnifies your style. When you have one, look for another.

Although high fashion garments are exhilarating, shrewd shoppers manage to build a chic wardrobe using good budget sense and all discount and sales options. Consistency in taste is possible at any price level. Interchangeable and coordinating outfits offer multiple choices with economy. We don't need lots of clothes when we have mixables.

I seldom see the husbands of clients, but I did meet two whose wives were surprisingly similar. Harriet is in her mid-50s and Susan, just over 60. Both have been married for 30 or more years, and it was obvious their spouses still admire them. These women have cheerful dispositions with sunny smiles, a zest for life and pride in appearance that is not the least bit egotistic – all on a modest budget.

This does not suggest that beauty-consciousness is the solution to matrimonial bliss. Far from it! But, for centuries women have known they must nurture appearance with more care than men do. No woman knew this better than Queen Elizabeth I of England. During her reign in the 1500s, she wanted to impress, influence, be remembered and loved by her people. She portrayed herself as a caring monarch in appearance as much as anything, and it was no accident. She planned it that way and wanted it that way up to her last breath. Many modern women who are over fifty and very visible in the media and public life are repeating the same philosophy. They are practicing the principles of ageless beauty.

Putting our best look forward is essential to squeezing every ounce of satisfaction out of life. Being a lovely presence adds pleasure to our world, just as the fragrance of each blossom from the delicate wild flower to the exquisite rose whispers a note of joy to the beholder.

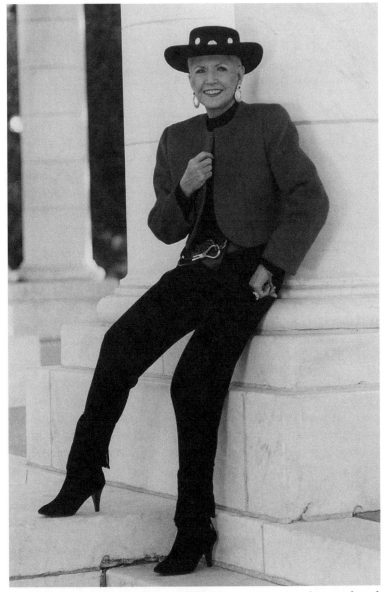

Betty Reed, a runway fashion model for over 40 years, has perfected the art of expressing the winning image through care, color and style. She has had two facelifts and may get another when she is 70. Diving and snorkeling in Mexico are her favorite sports. At 68, she passed the test to be a certified diver.

What message do you get
When you contemplate
A lovely little flower?
Be like me,
Make beauty a part of your life.
                    Leonard Andrews
                    *New York Daily News*[3]

Catherine Ponder in *The Prospering Power of Love*[4] tells of a way to create beauty, "You can glorify your own appearance and that of your world by creating as much beauty as possible. A famous actress was once asked how she stayed so young, though she was actually past 70. Her reply was that she remained youthful by looking at beauty, appreciating beauty, thinking about beauty.

"You can have more beauty in your world if you will begin right where you are to add whatever touches of beauty are possible. As you do this, beauty will multiply in your life. As you dwell more and more on beauty and do all that is possible to produce it in your world, you will become more successful and prosperous."

Katherine Hepburn[5] said she was glad to have been born a woman. "I think women are nicer. Don't you?" Think of all the parts women play in one lifetime – loving companion, mother, wife, grandmother, comforter, confidante, teacher, clubwoman, volunteer, provider, church worker, homemaker, storekeeper, businesswoman, artist, professional. The list goes on and on. While filling many roles simultaneously, women endure unbelievable hardships that would stymie many a stalwart male, yet they keep plugging along, often forgetting their own needs in favor of another's.

So, it's right to appreciate ourselves, to view ourselves compassionately, not critically. Self-depreciation accomplishes nothing. Passing middle age is a signal for new beginnings and happenings. If bulges or wrinkles can't be corrected, so what? Stop worrying about them. Use the fashion tips in this book. It's okay to have wrinkles and bulges. They're part of growing up! Beauty has many faces and forms. Youth is one; maturity is another – but with deeper meaning and the potential to rival youth. The youth ethic is okay, but the ageless ethic is better.

Many times we look better than we realize. We have a bad habit of listening to a personalized putdown syndrome. As I was waiting to interview a doctor for this book, I talked to his receptionist. Her silver-grey hair was smoothly coiffed and framed an openly friendly face with soft makeup colorings. She wore a two-piece grey knit suit flecked with green and turquoise that typified not age or youth but timeless style. When I told her she looked lovely, she exclaimed with genuine surprise, "Oh my, do I really?" Then she stood up and said, "But, just look at how fat I am!" She thought plumpness was a negative. A couple years after our meeting she had a facelift and breast reduction. These big ticket procedures gave her a sense of youthfulness she thought she lost and eliminated self-depreciation. She truly looked at least 15 years younger and loved the lighter body feeling. Sometimes it takes radical positive changes to create the life we are happy living. In her case, it was worth every dollar.

Living longer, actively and healthier is the trend of this era, and how we define appearance as well as the way we spend our time is important. In this context, birthdays don't count. Denouncing limiting self-talk, often caused by the critical tapes that creep in from a judgmental society, is not enough. We must cultivate positive expectancy, automatically questioning the legitimacy of the negative. It takes mental strength to exercise this wisdom, but the result is a contented and rewarding experience. Life need not be a waiting game. It can be an adventure in continual learning, creativity, enjoying health-giving activity and people, work, and service.

And, oh yes, SMILE. The loveliest you shines through the window of your smile. It's the best advertisement for the person you are and your passport to receiving more of what's rightfully yours continuing happiness, fulfillment and well-being.

# Notes

## Introduction

[1]Davis, Julie, *The Allure Book*, New York: Bantam Books, 1984, p.8

## Chapter 1
### The Magic of Color

[1]Marshall Editions Ltd. of London, *Color*, Los Angeles: The Knapp Press, 1980, p.10

[2]Itten, Johannes, *The Art of Color*, London: Van Norstrand Reinhold Co., 1973, p.16

[3]Gerson, Joel, *Standard Book for Professional Estheticians*, Bronx, NJ: Milady Publishing Corp., 1984, p.380

[4]Birren, Faber, *Color Psychology and Color Therapy*, Secaus, NJ: Citadel Press, 1961, p.xiii.

## Chapter 2
### The Basics

[1]Kerr, Jean, "Mirror, Mirror on the Wall, I Don't Want to Hear One Word Out of You," *The Snake Has All the Lines*, 1960.

[2]Gerson, Joel, *Standard Book for Professional Estheticians*, Bronx, NY: Milady Publishing Corp., 1984, p.204.

[3]Alexander, Dale, *Dry Skin and Common Sense*, West Hartford, CT: Witkower Press, Inc., 1978, p.63.

[4]Simon, M.D., Harvey B., *Conquering Heart Disease*, NY: Little, Brown, 1994, p.145.

[5]Brown, Michele and Anne O'Connor, *Hammer and Tongues*, NY: St. Martin's Press, Inc.

[6]Reilly, Harold J. and Ruth Hagy Brod, *The Edgar Cayce Handbook for Health,* Virginia Beach, VA: A.R.E. Press, 1975, p.289.

[7]Ibid., p.289.

[8]Ray, Tony, Angela Hynes, *The Silver/Grey Beauty Book,* NY: Rawson Associates, 1987.

[9]Carnegie, Dale, *How to Win Friends and Influence People,* NY: Pockets, 1982, p.66.

[10]Landers, Ann, *Gems* booklet, Chicago, IL: 1988, p.58.

[11]*Vogue* magazine, October, 1986.

[12]Bruce, Jeffrey, Sherry Cohen, *About Face,* NY: Pubnam Publishing Group, 1984, p.130.

[13]Linda Fang, M.D. is one of the first clinical dermatologists to put a non-chemical sunscreen into moisturizers and foundations.

## Chapter 3
### Be Your Own Makeup Artist

[1]Rubinstein, Helena, *My Life For Beauty,* NY: Simon & Schuster, 1966.

[2]Bruce, Jeffrey, Sherry Cohen, *About Face,* NY: Pubnam Publishing Group, 1984, p.129.

[3]*Ibid.,* p.129.

[4]Davis, Julie, *The Allure Book,* NY: Bantam Books, 1984, p.94.

[5]*Porter Hospital Newspaper,* Denver, CO, Spring 1987.

## Chapter 4
### You Can Brighten Your Smile!

[1]Viorst, Judith, *Forever Fifty,* NY: Simon & Schuster, 1989, p.49.

[2]Modern Maturity, *Braces – At My Age?,* September-October 1987, p.27.

[3]Senior World, Los Angeles, CA, May 1990.

## Chapter 5
### Erasing the Wrinkles and Breast Reduction

[1]*Senior Spotlight,* Denver, CO, April 1989, p.15.
[2]*Facts for Consumers, Cosmetic Surgery,* Federal Trade Commission, Office of Consumer/Business Education, Washington, D.C., March 1990.
[3]Maltz, Dr. Maxwell, *Pscho-Cybernetics,* p.152.

## Chapter 6
### Where is Your Hair Headed?

[1]Jacobson, Carlotta Karlson, *How to be Wrinkle-Free,* NY: Putnam Publishing Group, 1986, p.115.
[2]Robertson, Laurel, Carol Flinders, Bronwen Godfrey, *Laurel's Kitchen,* Petaluma, CA: Bantam/Nilgiri Press, 1978, pp.430, 448-450.
[3]Gerson, Joel, *Standard Textbook for Professional Estheticians,* p.176.

## Chapter 7
### Fashion for Your Figure

[1]Warner, Carolyn, *The Last Word, a Treasury of Women's Quotes,* Englewood Cliffs, NJ: Prentice Hall, Inc., 1992, p.274.

## Chapter 8
### Hands

[1]Bozic, Patricia, *30 Days to Beautiful Nails,* NY : Warner Books, 1984, p.64.
[2]Arpel, Adrien, *851 Fast Beauty Fixes and Facts,* NY: Warner Books, 1984, p.64.
[3]NeoStrata's AHA Gel For Age Spots lightens discolorations. Call 1-800-865-8667 for more information
[4]Bozic, *30 Days to Beautiful Nails,* pp.11,18.

## Chapter 9
### Accessories

[1]*Senior Focus,* Bremerton, WA, December 1990.

## Chapter 10
### Restoring a Positive Image After Mastectomy and Ileostomy

[1]Hjelmstad, Lois Tschetter, *Fine Black Lines, Reflections on Facing Cancer, Fear and Loneliness,* Denver, CO: Mulberry Press, p.160.
[2]One non-chemical, inert ingredient is titanium dioxide, used as a physical barrier to block a broad spectrum of UV radiation. The Linda Sý Non-Chemical Sunscreen SPF 16 is available from dermatologists or call 1-800-232-3376 in California and 1-800-422-3376 outside California.

### Epilogue
### Birthdays Don't Count!

[1]Whitman, Walt, *Leaves of Grass,* NY: W. W. Norton & Co., 1860, p.275.
[2]*Vogue* magazine, June 1987.
[3]*Newsweek* magazine, August 18, 1986.
[4]Ponder, Catherine, *The Prospering Power of Love,* Marina Del Rey, CA: Devorss and Company, 1983, p.64
[5]*Ladies Home Journal,* October 1987.

# Bibliography

Alexander, Dale, *Dry Skin and Common Sense*, West Hartford, CT: Witkower Press, Inc., 1978.

Begoun, Paula, *Don't Go to the Cosmetics Counter Without Me*, WA: Beginning Press, 1996.

Begoun, Paula, *Don't Go Shopping for Hair Care Products Without Me*, WA: Beginning Press, 1995.

Berger, Karen and John Bostwick III, M.D., *A Woman's Decision Breast Care, Treatment, and Reconstruction*, New York: The C. V. Mosby Company, New York, 1994.

Birren, Faber, *Color Psychology and Color Therapy*, Secaus, NJ: Citadel Press, 1961.

Buchanan, Sue Love, *Laughter & a High Disregard for Statistics*, Nashville, TN: Thomas Nelson Publishers, 1994.

Burns, George, *How to Live to Be 100 or More*, G. P. Putnam's Sons, New York, 1983.

Cameron, Julia, *The Artist's Way*, G. P. Putnam's Sons, New York, 1992.

Carnegie, Dale, *How to Win Friends and Influence People*, New York: Pocket Books, 1982.

Gerson, Joel, *Milady's Standard Book for Professional Estheticians*, Bronx, New York: Milady Publishing Corp.

Hill, Napoleon, *The Law of Success*, Chicago, IL: Success Unlimited, Inc., 1979.

Hjelmstad, Lois Tschetter, *Fine Black Lines*, Denver, CO: Mulberry Hill Press, 1993.

Maltz, Dr. Maxwell, *Psycho-Cybernetics*, New York: Simon & Schuster, 1960.

Ponder, Catherine, *The Prospering Power of Love*, Marina Del Rey, CA: Devorss and Company, 1983.

Reilly, Harold J. and Ruth Hagy Brod, *The Edgar Cayce Handbook for Health Through Drugless Therapy*, Virginia Beach, VA: A.R.E. Press, 1975.

Simon, Harvey B., M.D., *Conquering Heart Disease*, NY: Little, Brown, 1994.

Stone, Justin F., *T'ai Chi Chih!*, San Luis Obispo, CA: Satori Resources, 1987.

Viorst, Judith, *Forever Fifty*, New York, New York: Simon and Schuster, 1989.

Yanker, Gary and Kathy Burton, *Walking Medicine*, McGraw-Hill, 1993.

U.S. Department of Health and Human Services, *Physical Activity and Health*, A Report of the Surgeon General, Washington D.C.: 1996, to order write Superintendent of Documents, P.O. Box 371954, Pittsburgh, PA 15250-7954

Warner, Carolyn, *The Last Word, a Treasury of Women's Quotes*, Englewood Cliffs, New Jersey: Prentice Hall, Inc., 1992.

Winter, Ruth, *A Consumer's Dictionary of Cosmetic Ingredients*, NY: Crown, (latest edition).

# Index

# W

## *Look Like A Winner After 50 With Care, Color & Style* is a thoughtful gift for the modern woman

Cost, $15.95 – Check your local bookstore, call credit card orders to 800-833-9327, or mail check/money order payable to
Golden Aspen Publishing
P.O. Box 370333, Denver, CO 80237-0333.

Shipping:  Book Rate $2.00; Priority Mail $3.50

Colorado Sales Tax:  Please add $1.16 sales tax if shipped to a Denver County address; outside Denver County but in Colorado, add 61 cents.

### Golden Aspen Publishing offers these special reports for cost-conscious women:

See a Glowing Face with Easy Daily Care
Alpha Hydroxy Products Help Your Skin to Be Smooth
Be Your Own Makeup Artist!
Where is Your Hair Headed?
How to Shop, Save and Select Clothing for your Figure
Beauty Tips for Breast Cancer Survivors
How to Restore a Positive Image After Mastectomy

### – New reports not based on the book –

A Smorgasbord of Ideas to Help you Stay Up to Date
Why Not Have an Almost New Face? (laser resufacing)
100+ Ways to Win the Age Game
Pump Up Your Body, Mind, & Spirits with Planned Physical Activity – 27 Reasons to Go for it and 10 Easy Exercises

**Write GAP, phone 303-694-6555, or fax 303-694-0737 for your free copy of our catalogue.**